Laurie's Journey

Love Always Wins

Linda L. Jones

Copyright © 2013 Linda L. Jones
All rights reserved.

All Bible verses in this book are taken from:
THE HOLY BIBLE, NEW INTERNATIONAL VERSION®, NIV® Copyright © 1973, 1978, 1984, 2011 by Biblica, Inc.® Used by permission. All rights reserved worldwide.

ISBN: 1492252697
ISBN-13: 978-1492252696

Library of Congress Control Number: 2013916663
CreateSpace Independent Publishing Platform
North Charleston, South Carolina

Introduction

I never set out to write a book. I'm a boring person who makes a living in the world of insurance. But it was not how I made my living, but how I made my *life* that prompted me to start setting down the words that eventually became this book.

It didn't start out to be a book, though. It began as a series of emails to let family and friends know our devastating news: that my beautiful partner, Laurie Roth—the other half of my soul, the one who completed my world just by stepping into it—had been diagnosed with breast cancer.

When you are in the fight of your life, the last thing you're thinking about is "Hey, maybe I'll make a book out of this." When the gloves are on and the dukes are up, it's really tricky to hold a pen or type an email. But what Laurie and I quickly realized was that we were not alone. We had our family and friends standing right beside us, praying for us on most days, loving us on all days. We had an army of people anxiously awaiting every phone call, every text, every email. So as Laurie's battle with cancer continued, we kept friends and family updated about her progress through emails and eventually through a blog. Laurie was far too humble to write about herself. So I, Linda—her partner, sidekick, and greatest fan—counted it my privilege and honor to tell her story. It was through those emails and blog posts, Laurie's amazing courage, and the love of our army that this book began to take shape.

As I wrote and shared and reached out, what I was really doing was telling a story. Our story. Laurie's and mine. My favorite story of all. It's a story of two people who met seemingly by chance, fell in love, and quickly realized that this love was heaven-sent. It's a story of two people whose souls were so intertwined from the get-go that it was as if we were one. It's a story of two people who

Linda L. Jones

continue to be tethered at our heartstrings, even though we've been divided from each other physically. In short, it's a love story. Our love story.

Sharing it now with more than just friends and family seems right. Allowing more people to know the amazing Laurie Roth will always be right. Praying that it helps even one person, one couple, or one family not only seems right, it *is* right. It's the way Laurie lived—to serve, to make life easier for others, to make this world a better place. She did that every day of her life, through sickness and in health. May this book carry on Laurie's beautiful traditions of grace under fire, inspirational living, and unconditional love.

Prologue

Laurie's journey began in May 2008. That was the first time we heard the devastating words "You have breast cancer." Those are words that truly knock you to your knees. They are the sucker punch that you never see coming. You certainly never expect it, especially if you are Laurie Roth, the healthiest, strongest, most I-can-do-absolutely-anything person I had ever met. You certainly never expect that sucker punch if you are me, Linda Jones. After all, I had been enjoying life basking in Laurie's beauty, inside and out, watching her be a hero to me and to so many others, thankful and proud to be her sidekick for life. No, those are the words that take your wonderful life and throw it directly into the spin cycle.

If you would indulge me just a bit, I'd like to tell you a little about our wonderful life. We were blessed from the get-go, knowing we found the other half of each other's heart. And we owed it all to my little cocker spaniel, Max Jones. It was Maxie that took off from me one day at a dog park, seemingly in search of a blowing leaf, a butterfly, or anything else that may have caught his short attention span. Oh, how I had sold that boy short. He knew exactly what he was doing, where he was going, and for whom he was looking.

He was especially determined on this run. I tried to keep up with him, but since I don't even run to the mailbox, it wasn't easy. His little legs were carrying him fast and furious. After he rounded a clump of trees, I lost sight of him and yelled his name. Just as I was getting to the trees, I heard the softest voice say, "Well, hello there." I came around the trees and found Max sitting, seemingly obedient, right at the feet of the most beautiful woman I had ever laid my eyes on. He was staring up at her with his little tail wagging and wiggling, so excited at his find. Laurie was staring down at him, smiling her gorgeous Laurie Roth smile, smitten with the little imp in front of her. I was trying to catch my breath, no longer just from running, but from being in the presence of an angel who had completely taken my breath away. Maxie looked over at me with a look on his face that said it all: "I found her, Mom, and I want to keep her." So keep her we did.

And in keeping her close, we found ourselves with one of the kindest, sweetest, most loving people ever created. And when Laurie Roth tucked you in her heart and kept you, you found heaven on earth. It was paradise found for both of us. Magical. Extraordinary. Soul mates. Once-in-a-lifetime love. Those aren't just my words, they are the words of so many who knew us, walked with us, loved us through our journey. We truly never took for granted that we had been given an incredible gift when Max brought us together. We not only found each other, we found the other half of each other's heart and a love that lives on and cannot be separated.

To indulge me just a bit more, let me tell you about this Laurie Roth. She was a special education teacher for twenty-eight years in our local school district. Her deep commitment and dedication to her students only made me love her more. It was a privilege to watch her touch the lives of her students, their families, and her peers. Hers was a life of service and of caring for others as often as she could. She developed reading programs that brought two of our dogs to schools to have children read to them, since she knew that children sitting in front of a dog felt safe enough to mispronounce a word, stumble through a sentence, or sound a word out loud to droopy ears. She gave her personal phone number to parents long before that became the norm, knowing that sometimes eight o'clock at night might be the only time parents would have time to chat about their concerns and worries. She knew that an involved parent was a good one to have around. They knew that Laurie was the kind of teacher they had hoped their children would have in their lives.

Beyond her teaching, she was the director of a pet therapy program that took dogs to area nursing homes. Even during her cancer treatment, Laurie rarely missed a pet therapy appointment. She would remind me that the residents might not have anyone else to visit them and that they would be waiting for us. So off we would go, Laurie exhausted and weak, but lighting up every room

Laurie's Journey

with her smile. Without fail, the exhausted and the weak we were visiting always smiled back.

If you're detecting a theme that pets were a focal point in Laurie's life, you are absolutely right. That's just something else we had in common. Pets have been the center of our lives, and we were always all the better for them. Maxie, our little matchmaking cocker spaniel, had been my dog initially but soon became Laurie's little man. I was there to give him treats and lend a lap, but it was Mama Laurie who hung the moon for him, just like she hung the moon for me. Our pets have also included two golden retrievers, Journey and Harbour; an ornery, bossy, loyal-to-a-fault cat named Ali; and a young cat named Hobo that Laurie found and insisted we take into our fold. All of our pets had one Alpha—Laurie—and one Omega—me. They knew that Laurie was in charge and often confused me for a littermate. Somehow we made it work and formed a family filled with love and joy and so much laughter.

Beyond family and friends known lovingly as Laurie's Lifesavers, some secret weapons up in heaven stayed on the journey with us. They included Laurie's grandparents on both sides, who adored their girl on earth and love her still from heaven; my mom, who loved Laurie from the minute she met her, often siding with her, much to my chagrin; and eventually our little Max. We lost him far too soon, but his big spirit remained tucked inside our hearts and every corner of our home.

Together, we became a pretty unbeatable team. Yet when we heard the words "You have breast cancer" in May 2008, we were shell-shocked, world-rocked, and very nearly paralyzed. Well, I should say that I was very nearly paralyzed. Laurie? Not so much. Laurie stood up, seeming even taller than usual. In Laurie's mind these were fighting words, and they brought out the fighter in her. After all, cancer was messing with Laurie's life, Laurie's world, Laurie's journey. A life, a world, a journey of hope, of courage, and certainly of love. And on this journey, love always wins.

I said earlier that Max and I kept Laurie. The honest truth is that she kept us.

PART 1

Treatment Begins

Laurie Doesn't Lose
July 16, 2008

We met with the oncologist, Dr. M., this afternoon to discuss treatments. So far Laurie has endured countless scans, blood tests and procedures, including a lumpectomy, a lymph node biopsy and most recently a bronchoscopy. To no one's surprise, she muscled through these like she's always done—brave-faced, courageously, and calmly. I almost had to be sedated just hearing about the procedures, but that is a story for another time (and comes to no surprise to anyone either). Unfortunately the bronchoscopy was basically inconclusive as to whether or not one stray lymph node was benign or malignant. Since we already know that other malignant nodes exist, we decided to forgo additional surgical procedures.

So, to make a long story short, we have made the decision, armed with much knowledge from Dr. M. and much research on our part, to move forward with a regimen of chemo treatment. Laurie will begin systemic chemotherapy on July 30th. Her treatments will more than likely consist of four rounds of chemo, once every three weeks.

There are other courses of chemo treatments, but Dr. M. feels Laurie is a very good candidate for the four round one. In addition to being fewer in number, it also has less of an overall impact on her heart. After the course of chemo is complete, they will do another PET scan and see where things stand. If everything is clear, she will begin a hormone treatment--it will consist of a pill every day for five years, as well as close testing and blood work.

We believe, as does Dr. M., that the chemo will not only take care of the breast cancer, but also if this stray node was actually malignant, it will take care of that too.

I personally believe that we need to get Laurie in the fight. We've waited and tested and waited some more, all the while allowing time to pass and anxiety to grow. The treatment plan coupled with her powerful determination, will conquer this. Cancer doesn't know this yet, but Laurie doesn't lose. Period. Once she is able to put her heart, mind and soul in it, cancer will be no match for Laurie.

That is not to minimize the emotions that go along with the diagnosis of breast cancer and all that is required for the fight. It's scary, it makes you sick, you probably lose your hair, and the list goes on and on. She can do it, but we are glad that we have you with us. Please keep her in your prayers and your thoughts, as you have already. You are all our lifelines and we are so blessed to have each of you in the fight with us.

Our Burly Angel
July 30, 2008

One round of chemo down, three more to go (God willing)! Today we started on the road to really beating this cancer thing. Laurie endured her first chemo like the champ that she is. And while we know that this treatment can take its toll as it progresses, we feel good having one round done.

We arrived at the Community Cancer Center at 8:30 a.m., anxious, nervous, scared—you name the apprehensive emotion and we probably had it. After the lab work was completed, we were taken back to the chemo chairs. We were now looking out windows we had only ever looked in. The cancer center is just a few blocks from our house, and for years we have walked the dogs around the windows and around the grounds. All those years of seeing other people in the chairs, and now one of us was in one.

Anyway, we soon found out that angels come in all shapes and sizes. We had been there only a few minutes when a burly type of guy and his wife came in. He was placed in the chair next to Laurie's. He seemed gruff, very rough around the edges, and I worried that this might make the day even longer. How wrong I was. His name is Skip, and he is a retired construction worker who has cancer of the throat, but a heart of gold.

Within minutes, Skip was showing us the ropes, pointing out which nurses are best at putting in IVs, explaining how to work the TV, and encouraging us to buy a DVD player to pass the time. He gave us tips and pointers we would never have known. His smile lit up his face and, in turn, lit up ours. More than anything else Skip showed us or taught us, he made us realize that you can laugh during chemo. His sense of humor helped get us through.

Believe me, laughing was really the last thing we thought we would be doing today—but God knew it should be one of the first. So He sent Skip to greet us on our first day. And laugh we did. Forever we will be thankful for this angel, this burly angel in cut-off jeans watching DVDs of pro wrestling, named Skip.

We go back next week for an appointment with Dr. M., and then the next chemo is slated for August 22. Until then, we pray that the side effects are minimal and for the strength to meet them head on. We are scared of the unknown, and yet I know the strength that is in Laurie. She can do it, there's no doubt in my mind. But these will be tough months ahead. And when we win, we will have a lifetime of months to enjoy.

There Must Be a Plan
September 12, 2008

We were never told that this whole chemo thing would be a fun ride. After all, it's chemo, not Children's Tylenol. We knew this would take every ounce of courage and strength that could be mustered up. Each round brings its own surprises of side effects, as well as the old ones from the past. In the world of chemo, familiarity really does breed contempt.

It's difficult to embrace chemo, even though it's saving your life. It's really hard to welcome it with open arms when it's tearing your body apart. It's tough to make it your friend when this is the "friend" that took your hair, makes you sick, and leaves you weak as a kitten. There are times when you truly question which side chemo is fighting for. Who needs friends like that? Unfortunately, this time, we do. Because Laurie and chemo are the one-two punch that will beat this thing.

As of today, we have three rounds down and one to go. This is a journey not for weaklings, which is why Laurie is often seen carrying me. Her stamina, her bravery, her unflinching will to face this head on are humbling and awe-inspiring all at the same time. This chemo is the toughest around. It has hurricane strength as it races through your body, fighting so hard to give you your life back, chasing and destroying those nasty cancer cells. But chemo can't discriminate, and it takes your good cells with it too. And those are the guys you really need right now. The weapons you would normally have to fight the fight with are erased, leaving it up to just you and chemo.

But it's Laurie, and she doesn't know how not to win. Cancer is quite the foe, though, and hits her with some really tough stuff;

Laurie's Journey

Laurie says, "That's your best?" and keeps on going. The "cure" causes problems and pains and anxiety that would knock most people down, and they would stay down; Laurie says, "I must stay standing," and she not only stands, but gets up and gets moving. The whole rotten process has tried to take her dignity, her identity, and makes giving in seem like a really good option; Laurie says, "This will not beat me," and keeps on fighting. Laurie's in the fight; cancer's going down.

So here come the tough weeks. History tells us that she'll be sick and weak and so very tired from about the second day of treatment through about the fourteenth or fifteenth. She'll then have five or six good days, and she lives every minute of them. The mere thought of having to endure the treatment would be enough to make most people want to throw in the towel. At the very least, most would whine and cry and wonder why this was happening. Not Laurie. Someone asked her, "Don't you ever wonder—why you?" Laurie's reply? "No. Why wouldn't it be me? Why would it be anyone else?"

She worries about our pal Skip, from the first round of chemo, and Lloyd, from the second round. Lloyd is an eighty-year-old guy who lost his wife of sixty years just a few weeks before his first treatment for prostate cancer. Laurie constantly reminds me that there are people worse off than us and that everyone has their challenges; this one just happens to be ours. There will be no pity parties in this house, except for the ones that I secretly throw for myself when Laurie isn't looking. There are others to worry about, others to care about, and others that need our good thoughts and deeds. That's Laurie in a nutshell.

Me? Off the top of my head, I can reel off a hundred names that I think should be tested like this, have their world rocked, get to worry what's coming next. I could keep naming names, including my own, and never, ever get to Laurie. She is one of God's angels, teaching us all how to live this life, how to treat others, how to be the change we want to see in this world. I admit that it is me, late at night when sleep won't come but worry sits right by my side, who has been known to whisper, "Why her, Lord, *why her*? Didn't you mean to pick someone else?"

And on those nights, I am reminded of a Babbie Mason song, "Trust His Heart." Its message is that God doesn't make mistakes, so we need to trust His plan even if we don't understand its purpose.

That's the hard part. We know that there must be a plan; we're just not privy to it. It may just be that God picks His best to show us how to do this thing called life. Who better than Laurie to show us grace under fire? Who better than Laurie to give love back when so many things have been taken from her? Who better than Laurie to keep walking, following the unknown path, until she arrives victoriously at the finish line we're shooting for?

And if that doesn't convince me and I spend far too much time worrying, God sends my mom into the game. She taps me—not so gently, I might add—and reminds me that we can do this, we're not alone. We have a secret weapon now in the guardian angel that is my mom. She arrived in heaven two weeks before Laurie's diagnosis. Laurie was one of my mom's all-time favorite people. In fact, Mom often favored Laurie over her own children, much to our chagrin. Mom was pretty powerful here on earth—I can only imagine what she can do from heaven. Between Laurie and my mom, cancer does not stand a chance. In fact, cancer might want to start running. You know what? I like that plan!

Close to the Finish Line
October 3, 2008

Before all the chemo started, when we were still in the planning stages, I read an article about a woman who ran 5Ks and 10Ks throughout her treatment. I remember thinking, "This will be Laurie." Even though she no longer runs, I knew she would be tempted to start up again just to show cancer who is in charge. I also knew that this would mean I would have to start running, and since I don't run to the mailbox, I knew I had to bring this idea to a screeching halt. I told Laurie that we would find other ways to stick it to cancer.

But run she has. She has run in her own way through this treatment. Not from cancer, not from chemo, not from anything. She is running to her finish line. Today, with her fourth and final treatment, she gets breathtakingly close to that finish line.

Be proud of this remarkable person that you call your daughter, your sister, your friend. She faced today with her usual grace and made it through with her usual array of flying colors.

Laurie enters the building with the same determination that gets her through the toughest of days, knowing full well this is one of them. I'm sure every fiber of her body is begging her to run the other way. I cannot look her in the eye, because in my eyes she would see tears. Knowing that her sidekick really needs to buck up, I act distracted, fumble around with the car keys and magazines, and make ridiculous small talk, all the while praying that this is the last leg of our race to find a cure and that we have left cancer in the dust.

We go in, and Laurie begins looking for all of our favorites. We look for Skip, knowing that his cancer is not shrinking, only growing in new places. Skip needs a couple of angels, just like he was ours at that first treatment that now seems so long ago. We smile at Lloyd, who quietly takes his chemo while reading the book by Randy Pausch, *The Last Lecture*. With our eyes brimming with tears, we say a prayer that Lloyd is nowhere near his last lecture. We look around, and Laurie reminds me that we are so much better off than many with whom we share this room.

Laurie's determination through all of this has been predicated on a plan that her life would remain as normal as possible. When her hair began falling out, when her hair was completely gone, when a wig and hats were her only options, she found life as usual somehow. When her body ached, when climbing a few stairs took all her strength, when her mouth broke out in merciless sores, she found her life as she once knew it. She knew that finding pieces of her old life would be her ticket out of this new one, and that was a perfect plan.

So she got up every day and went to school, because that was normal. She greeted her students with her beautiful smile that let them know that Miss Roth is just fine, and then so were they. She came home to Max and Journey, who have a routine of being walked within seven seconds of Laurie's arrival, and she dutifully went and got their leashes. She listened to my boring stories about insurance and my dull days and didn't use an ounce of strength to roll her eyes to the back of her head. She simply listened.

She knows that her students need to see her and see her smile. She knows that Max and Journey need her to walk with them. She knows that I need to tell her about my day and that it will be boring. She knows that in those brief moments, she's no longer in that other world, that other life. She is Laurie Roth, and it's her world and life as usual. In her heart, she prays that it soon will be.

Laurie's Journey

She is the epitome of courage. For the rest of my life, I will bask in the shadow of her grace, her strength, her peace. The easiest thing for her to do would have been to give up, give in, lie down. But those options never entered her brain. To look at this serene soul who brings calm to the chaos, you would never know the fighter that lurks within. As the old saying goes, "It's not the size of the dog in the fight, it's the size of the fight in the dog." The size of Laurie's fight is immeasurable. Laurie is fighting like her life depends on it. Laurie is fighting because she knows it does.

Round four is down and weaving through her body. The effects of chemo are cumulative, so this may add up to be the worst one yet. It will hurt her, she will have pain and constant discomfort, and it will make her wonder if this is the one that breaks her. If Laurie has a breaking point, I've not seen it. I'm sure she wishes she could say the same of me.

Where do we go from here? In a few short weeks, Laurie will have another body scan to see how things are looking. We are hopeful and confident that the one-two punch of Laurie and chemo have sent cancer flying. We ask for your continued support, your prayers, and all of your good thoughts as we wait for the good news that pushes us across the finish line. Then the true finish line of breast cancer will be to go five years cancer-free. We're shooting for the five-year mark; we're shooting for a lifetime.

We know that God does nothing randomly. And while there are lesser things He could have chosen Laurie for, He is showcasing this angel for a reason. A reason that we may know someday, or a reason that we may never know. But we do know of a favorite Bible verse, Jeremiah 29:11, in which God says, "For I know the plans I have for you . . . plans to prosper you and not to harm you, plans to give you hope and a future." That's all we're asking for, and I pray that's what we get—hope and a future. There's no end to what we can do with that.

You, as our lifelines, have made all the difference in this race. God's blessings come not just in the strength that He brings to Laurie, but in the love He gives from you. Please never underestimate the power of your love, your smiles, your cards, and your thoughts. Laurie is buoyed by all of you; we are blessed with each of you.

Joy Comes in the Morning
October 28, 2008

We went today for the results of Laurie's biopsy. As you know, while the overall PET scan results were very good and showed no evidence of cancer in most of her body, there was a rogue lymph node that was concerning. That lymph node was biopsied last week, and today we were told that it was positive for cancer.

While we would have loved to hear that it was negative and that all was good, we are thankful that it was caught. Right now, one lymph node is controllable, one lymph node can be removed, one lymph node may even be able to be radiated and blasted out of there. But if one lymph node were to go undetected, it could undo all that chemo and Laurie fought so hard for. It could move to other lymph nodes, it could move to other parts of her body, and it could cause many problems that we don't even dare to think about. So we thank God that it was found and that we can take care of it now, not chase it later.

We asked both the oncologist and the radiology oncologist: Why did chemo not get this? They both explained that due to the extent of Laurie's surgeries to that area, the blood supply was cut off, allowing this lymph node to remain, and chemo could not get to it. Chemo moves through systemically, protecting the body from the spread of cancer. The PET scan confirms that the chemo was successful. The lymph node involved was not exposed to chemo; therefore it remains. Not a common occurrence, but it happens.

We so wanted to be done with all of this. I doubt you could find two people more eager to start radiation—it clearly shows that we need to get a life, if this is the kind of stuff we look forward to! But it looks like we are going on a little detour first. We've yet to take a road trip without one, so why should this be different? Our detour will probably come in the form of one more surgery to remove the lymph node. We're gathering some additional opinions, but we are leaning toward just getting that thing out of there. The doctors aren't able to tell us with utmost certainty that if we only do radiation, then radiation could get it all. They think it "probably" could. Laurie's life deserves an answer that is more than a "probably"; Laurie's life deserves a "you'd better believe we will get it!" Surgery provides that answer.

The surgery will probably take place within a few weeks and hopefully not be that invasive. It will involve making an incision in the same general area of her prior surgeries, removing the lymph node, and closing her up. Approximately three to four weeks later, her radiation will begin. The good news of surgery plus radiation: Laurie's chances of recurrence dramatically drop. And that's what we're shooting for.

I think everyone will agree with me when I say that Laurie Roth is a unique person, one of a kind, with no duplication. I'm convinced God made just one of her because one would be more than enough for this world to enjoy. You don't get more special than Laurie. While we are more than ready for God to move His spotlight to someone else, we are so very thankful that we have options, that there is a "you'd better believe we will get it" answer, that the light at the end of the tunnel continues to glisten for us.

There is a Bible verse (Psalm 30:5) that says, "Weeping may stay for the night, but rejoicing comes in the morning." We have been in the midst of a pretty dark night, and there have been tears, many tears—some falling right now, mainly from sheer exhaustion and disbelief. Today we wanted to see the bright rays of sunshine signaling that our morning was here. As tired as Laurie is, as much as she deserves to see her morning, as much as we hoped that our joy would come today, we will wait for the arrival of the joy we know is coming.

That morning will be celebrated with the exuberance generally confined to Super Bowls, the births of babies, and soldiers coming home. That morning will be filled with uproarious laughter, smiles that won't be able to leave our faces, and probably even some tears, but these will be tears of pure joy. That morning is close, the race is nearly done, and Laurie is more than ready for her victory lap. She'll run that lap, she'll have that morning, she'll have that celebration. More important, she'll have a lifetime. And right then, we will all know the joy that we have been promised.

Merry Christmas 2008
December 25, 2008

On this day, we are reminded of the many blessings that we have in our lives. If you are receiving this email, you are certainly one of them, one that we are so very thankful for.

Laurie's Journey

Christmas is a time that reminds us of all that is good in this world. A time that shows us that despite the heartache, despite the fears, and despite all that seems wrong, there is much that is right, much that returns pure joy, and so much that gives us hope. And as we have mentioned in the past, you can do anything when you have hope.

It is no secret that this has been a year that gave us much reason to pause, to reflect, to take stock in all that was right in our world. It was a year that knocked us to our knees not once, but twice. Once with my Mom's death and then again, two weeks later, with Laurie's breast cancer diagnosis. Both brought pain, pain that at times seemed intolerable. Both brought tears, tears that seemed unceasing. And both brought fear, a fear of "where do we go from here," because "here" didn't seem like the best starting point. It all seemed too much to bear.

But when knocked to your knees, you have a couple of choices. You either stay down or look up. Since Laurie won't let us stay down (as I am more than willing to do), she made us both look up. So we looked up and saw God looking down, ready to carry us, reminding us that He had this one and we could rest. We looked up and saw the light that reminds us that no matter how dark it is, we are not alone. And we looked up and saw you, each of you, with your hands reaching down and your arms outstretched and your heads nodding that this was one we would all face together.

You came in the form of phone calls and cards and flowers and plants. You came in the form of visits and dinners and prayers and smiles. You came and you made us laugh. You came and you let us cry. Simply put, you came. You came and you stayed. And we will be forever grateful.

So on this Christmas morning, we pray that you feel the same love from those in your life that make your spirits bright. The thought of you does that for us.

Right Around the Corner
January 25, 2009

We try to view life as a journey. In fact, after Taylor, our last dog, passed and we were desperately wondering how we would go on without her, we found a way to move forward through a little puppy, another golden retriever. We appropriately named her Journey, knowing full well that the torch had been passed and we would move on to the many more journeys in store for us. Life is an incredible journey, with high hills to climb, bumps in the road, and turns that you never saw coming. It is also a journey of joys too many to count, smiles and laughs shared by dear friends and special family, and sheer happiness from living life with those you love.

We know there will be days when we want to sing from the mountaintops, days when the valleys seem too low to bear, and days when we want to cry, maybe even wail a bit. We know that life gives you reasons to pause and reasons to count your blessings and reasons to keep going when everything around you says that you can't.

We've come to realize that life is the whole enchilada—the good, the bad, the ugly. It is living with cancer, it is living with chemo, it's living without your hair, it is living when life really is not one bit attractive. But you wake up and realize that it's the one shot you get and you'd better take it. We're not tested on the mountaintops when we're singing our hearts out. Our tests come in the valleys, over the bumps, and in turns you never saw coming.

Laurie's Journey

So you do what you do when faced with any turn in the road. If you're Laurie and you're smart, you turn. You turn because dead ends aren't in your vocabulary. You turn because the route you were going down wasn't the road you wanted to be on anyway. You turn, and you pray that the turn brings you out to a much better place.

But where to turn is the nagging question. And just when you need to, you know the answer. You turn to your inner strength, and you find that you still have some. You turn to your friends and your family, and they race to your side and renew you. You turn to God, and you are reminded of the strength and peace He holds out as His forever promise to you. And through each of these answers, you pray that you will soon be turning the corner.

That corner is close. We can see it, we can feel it, and we are so close to celebrating it. That corner comes on February 3, when Laurie gets her last radiation treatment. Radiation doesn't hold a candle to its cousin chemo, but it's no walk in the park either. It has burned her skin, it has hurt, and it has taken its own toll on her already beaten-up body. But in true Laurie fashion, she's been the shining example of how to face the unfaceable.

They said she would get tired, and she did. But when she was really tired, she took long walks behind Nurse Journey, who saw it as her duty to get Mommy's heart rate up—way up—and keep it up forty-five to fifty minutes later. (Max and I go for five or ten and then return completely exhausted to our Pepsi and Doritos.) They said that she wouldn't have much strength in her upper arm, and that was true. But when she thought it might even think about acting up, she reminded her body who was boss and went out and snowblowed five driveways. (I cheered her on from the living room.) They said that her skin would be raw, that it would peel and be painful, and it is. It is *really* painful. (I cry just looking at it.) But she dutifully puts her medicated cream on and faces the day anyway. Side effects really aren't in Laurie's game plan. They get in the way of life, and she will have none of that.

She is grace under fire, the poster child for bravery, and the calm in the chaos. She has rewritten the script on how to do this thing called life, taking the bumps and bruises as they come and finding a reason to smile anyway. Cancer scared her to the very depths of her soul, but it never once broke her. It pushed her to the very limits, but she pushed back. It tried to change her, but her heart and soul and beautiful spirit came out of this mess completely intact. As if she wasn't already, she cemented herself as my hero. And in my childlike mind, the hero always wins. In my heart of hearts, *this* hero has to win. And in my talks to God, He hears whispers that beg "Dear Lord, please let her win." This is the person meant to be on this earth, showing the rest of us how life works best when you do it right.

So what follows radiation? Laurie will have another scan in three to four months, when they are sure all of the radiation is out of her system. We are hopeful that we will then get our walking papers from this world of cancer. We are hopeful that the chemo and the radiation and the drug Tamoxifen are knocking cancer senseless and completely out of the park. We are hopeful that this hurdle has been jumped and the finish line is Laurie's for the taking.

And when we cross, we cross with each of you beside us, each of you cheering us on, each of you ready to celebrate. We thank you for your prayers, your good thoughts, and your love. We thank you for making this journey with us. Hang in there with us—we're so close. Keep praying, keep cheering, keep running. The celebration is right around the corner.

Holding Our Breath
March 15, 2009

The next step in this marathon will come on May 4, when Laurie has a CT scan. It's a period of time that's kind of a time out—let the dust settle and see where we're at in May. It's kind of scary, in a way, and freeing in another.

We have a plaque in our home that says, *"Life isn't measured by the number of breaths that you take but by the moments that take your breath away."*

We found it years ago in a store—accidentally stumbled into it, actually. We both thought it was a great way to think about life, so we bought it. We brought it home, hung it up, and smiled. "What a great saying!" we enthusiastically thought. At the time, we were equating this saying with only good times. We reminisced about those types of moments: when your heart is so full and you feel so great, and then all of a sudden, you are so happy that you absolutely cannot breathe. Hopefully, we all have had those moments.

Last May, we found that those moments come in the not-so-good times too. Last May, we heard the news that Laurie had breast cancer. When those words were spoken, when we actually heard them out loud, when my worst fear was realized, I can tell you that *that* is another moment that literally takes your breath away. It takes it so far away that you truly believe you will never breathe again. In many ways, I don't know that we have breathed the same since.

We've held our breath as we anxiously awaited test results and doctors' examinations. We've been short of breath from this tiring journey and emotional roller coaster. We've had our breath taken away with scares and worries, pain and heartache. And just when you think you will not, you cannot, there is absolutely no way you can take another breath, God whispers His hope into you, right where you need it, right when you need it, and holds your tired body and gives you strength. And just as He has promised, you do begin to breathe again.

The heart, too, is a funny thing and has a lot to do with this breathing thing. (I'm no anatomy major, but I think I'm right on this.) When our lives were changed forever, when we were told that Laurie has breast cancer, when the floor dropped completely out from under us, it seemed like our hearts stopped. I remember thinking, as the doctor was talking, that my heart was racing so fast I thought it might actually beat itself right out of my body. And yet, at the exact same time, I felt like it had stopped. Certainly, my world had.

Now, imagine Laurie's heart. She's just been told that she has breast cancer, she's just been told that she will have chemo, she's just been told that the cure to help her live will make her feel like she wants to die. Her breath had to be gone and her heart had to be stopped. Her heart had to be overwhelmed and overworked and probably pounding out of her shirt.

After all, this was not in the game plan. When you live life like Laurie, life is really good.

When you live life like Laurie, that's exactly what you do: you LIVE life. You're supposed to have countless journeys with Journey and constant laughs with our eternal child, Max.

You're supposed to have it be as good as it gets, because that's what she gives. It is supposed to have, it has to have, that "happily ever after," because if anyone's earned it, Laurie has.

Fortunately, God gave Laurie an incredible heart. Her heart beats so strongly that you can almost hear it when you sit next to her.

So when we got the word, while I was moving directly into the fetal position, she was moving on and moving forward. While I was replaying the words over and over in my mind, briefly paralyzed by the doctor's voice, Laurie was already standing up, actually standing stronger. While the tears rolled down my face and I could not utter one audible word, Laurie asked, "Where do we go from here?"—already anxious to get on with her life. I knew right then that cancer was not going to get in her way. I also knew that I was really going to have to buck up.

You see, as faithful as I try to be and as hopeful as I want to be, I have two very good friends named Anxiety and Worry. They're inconsiderate friends, because they tend to come for visits around 2:00 a.m. and stay until just before the alarm rings. They wake me up from a somewhat sound sleep, start the conversation off with a few "what ifs," throw in a couple of "uh-ohs," and when I'm completely wide-eyed, follow up with the ever dreaded "Here's one you might not have thought of." No wonder I'm barely breathing!

But Laurie, she sleeps. She must remember what Victor Hugo so eloquently reminds us: God is awake. She goes to sleep and stays asleep, knowing she will do what she can do and God will take it from there. She goes to sleep settled in her day and wakes up with even more determination than she started with the day before. She lives life with purpose. She lives life as gracefully and as courageously as anyone ever could. She is here to live, and nothing will get in her way.

Cancer certainly has tried, but it has never once won. I want the victory column to always read the same: Laurie Roth Wins, Cancer Loses. And as we sit here today, knowing that the next test is not until May 4, the one that will tell us that chemo did the trick, we sit here in what we call our "breathing room." It's the time between chemo and radiation, needle pricks and additional tests, doctors' visits and painful worries. It's the time that we are trying to enjoy, the time to breathe again, to live. It's the time to ask you once again to think good thoughts and say your prayers that Laurie will have breathing room for as long as she wants.

Our heartfelt thanks go out to each one of you who has held us in prayer, in thought, and in your heart. The Bible tells us that "and now these three remain: faith, hope and love. But the greatest of these is love" (1 Corinthians 13:13). May we all keep the faith that May 4 will bring the good news that we have waited for so long. May we all always have hope, because with hope you can do anything. And may we all have love like you have given us and like we hold so deeply for each of you.

We'll keep you posted. Get the horns ready—May 4 is the day we cross the finish line!

Race for the Cure
April 14, 2009

When we hatched this little idea to form a team for Peoria's Race for the Cure, Laurie and I never dreamed of the unbelievable turnout we would get. We told each other, "It's a tough weekend." "It's so early." "Even if we just have a few folks, that will still be fun." And then the names kept coming in, the roster kept filling up, until thirty people (and still counting) from our little world in Bloomington had signed up to go over to Peoria really early on a Saturday morning to race for the cure. Thank you!

I remember filling out the pages on the Komen site, and just for snicks, I set a team goal to raise one thousand dollars. I'm a

Laurie's Journey

simple person who thinks in simple ways and in round numbers. So a thousand dollars sounded good. I had no idea where it would come from and no thought whatsoever that we would come close to hitting it. I figured that when I handed in our team's pledge sheets, I'd sheepishly have to tell the race people, "We tried but fell a bit short." I thought it was better than "Hey, we tried. Do we still get the free T-shirt?"

After all, this was not about you going out and getting pledges. This was about us, teaming together, walking together, reminding Laurie that this was one walk she would never make alone. If we didn't raise one dime, Saturday, May 9 would still be a tremendous success.

Well, team, you knew far better than I did what we could do. Not only have we met the goal that I pulled completely out of the air, we've surpassed it. In fact, we have surpassed it by far. I am so excited to tell you that we are currently in fourth place!

And we have one more announcement. When we had this idea to bring our world to Peoria and all walk a mile with Laurie, I had to think of a name for our team. I thought so long and hard, my head hurt. (Okay, I thought for like five minutes, but my head really did hurt.) Remember, I'm a simple person who thinks in simple ways. I naturally went with the simple alliteration of Roth's Runners, even though this was a complete lie, since few of us had any intention of running.

So we thought maybe we could think of something better, a bit more apropos. And when I say "we could think of something better," I mean Shirley B. could think of something better. Shirley has by far one of the most creative minds ever made. I sent her an email begging her to brainstorm a name that sums us up, and to take her time, because I knew how tough a job it would be to get it just right. Seconds later, she emailed me back with a name so perfect, it still brings tears to my eyes when I think of it.

Shirley knows what everyone has meant to Laurie, and she made sure that the name reflected this. All of you have been Laurie's lifelines, her supporters, her whispers of hope and light in the darkest of moments. You have held her up when chemo made her weak, and you have stood tall with her when it could not knock her down. You have called, you have sent cards, you have sat by her and cried with her. You have cheered her on and held her hand, hugged her hard and softly prayed. You have been, and on May 9 you will officially be, Laurie's Lifesavers!

Hope and a Future
May 7, 2009

And everybody say "AMEN!"

I'm not sure what sounds you heard at 4:45 p.m. today, but in our world we heard four words that we were beginning to wonder if we would ever hear. Those four words? The four most beautiful words that I've heard in a long time. As we were holding our breath, barely brave enough to listen, we heard our favorite nurse say, "Laurie's scans look good." Read it and weep, folks. We did. We will for a long time. Weeping is definitely in order.

As is champagne popping, loud applause, dogs barking, and lots of hugs and smiles. These are the words that call for celebrations. These are the words that make the chemo, the radiation, the wigs, the sores, the aches and pains have meaning and purpose. These are the words that make today so worth waiting for. These are the words that clap Laurie on the back and say, "You did it, girl!"

And did she ever. With grace and courage, with humor and humility, with a brave smile and so few tears, she faced her foe. She not only faced it, she made it back down and cower. She took the toughest chemo, the longest radiation, and the hardest road imaginable and then sat for a few months wondering if all of that was going to be enough. Today, with just those four little words, she found out that it was ending up just right. In fact, "Laurie's scans look good" are about the most perfect words you will hear.

Something else that is about as perfect as we will ever know is you—each of you, with your outpouring of love and support, laughter and tears, and constant reminders that we would never take one single step alone. As lonely as this road could get, our road was filled with your footprints, your smiles, and your love. You made this marathon with us, and today you celebrate with us.

We mentioned awhile back a favorite Bible verse that reminds us that God's plan is to give us hope and a future. He made good on that promise today. For months, it seemed like we only had hope. And believe you me, there were days when I barely had that. I had worry, I had anxiousness, I had fear, I had fall-on-the-floor-and-wail. But hope? No. Hope could sometimes be a tough sale for me.

Yet right in front of me, God kept showing me Laurie. If that didn't point to hope and a future, I don't know what did. Each day she looked healthier, each day she seemed stronger, and each day she seemed farther away from cancer. Her smile got brighter, her steps got lighter, and there wasn't a single sign that she'd just walked through the fire. Could it be? Could I dare hope? Skeptically, I decided it was worth a shot. I decided that I'd close my eyes and take this leap of faith. I'd hope for the best and pray that our future would follow.

"Laurie's scans look good." If that doesn't have future written all over it, I don't know what does.

Thank you for being part of our past, our present, and our future. Thank you for everything.

The Climb
May 11, 2009

Since I won't be able to say it again until next year, this is your captain speaking, so please pay attention. This is also your captain at her humblest—so very thankful for each and every one of you who walked beside us and those that walked with us in spirit at Saturday's Race for the Cure.

May 9 had special significance long before Laurie's Lifesavers took form. Last year, on that exact date, I sat in a waiting room while Laurie underwent her first surgery for breast cancer. It was the surgery that would unequivocally tell us that our lives had just changed and we would never be the same again. I remember searching the surgeon's eyes, praying that I'd see his relief that the lump was not what we feared. Instead, he put his hand on my arm and said, "Let's hope for the best." A few days later, he gently told us that the lump was positive for breast cancer. I remember thinking that May 9 would go down as one of the worst days that I would ever know.

Fast forward to May 9, 2009. At a very early start time in Peoria, Illinois, bleary-eyed friends and family, now known as Laurie's

Laurie's Journey

Lifesavers, raced for the cure. You came in person and you came in spirit; and just like you have done throughout this year, you simply came. You came exactly when we needed you the most.

Laurie and I knew that we would do the Race for the Cure this year. We threw the idea out to you, and you bought it hook, line, and sinker, just like you've done every time we've even come close to uttering a need or a want. I can't imagine going through last year's May 9, this year's May 9, or any of the days in between without you.

We needed you there to walk with us, in person and in spirit, like you have so many times. I needed you there when I spied Laurie in the Survivors' Walk, and tears fell with the utter realization that my hero really had faced her foe and lived to tell about it. Laurie needed you as she took her place in this procession of survivors, her new comrades in arms, who had all faced, fought, and conquered their enemy. With all of us clapping, they walked to a song called "The Climb." Some special words from that song have incredible significance:

> *The struggles I'm facing*
> *The chances I'm taking*
> *Sometimes might knock me down*
> *but no, I'm not breaking . . .*
> *Ain't about how fast I get there*
> *Ain't about what's waiting on the other side*
> *It's the climb*

You've held Laurie through her struggles, you saw her get knocked down. But thanks to her awesome spirit bolstered by your love and support, not once did you see her break. She made that climb, *we* made that climb, with all of you cheering us on.

Saturday gave a whole new meaning to May 9. It's a day that Laurie's Lifesavers saved us again.

Unbelievable Spirit
February 13, 2010

Throughout Laurie's diagnosis, treatment, and recovery, we were often asked, "Do you have good support?"

We would just look at each other and smile. In terms of support, we knew we were covered. In fact, to refer to it as "good" was an understatement. So we often said, "Well, we don't have *good* support. We have absolutely unbelievable support." Last night was just one more beautiful example of the support that we have been blessed to have through each of you.

When we tell you that we couldn't have done it without you, we mean every word. This is a journey that if walked alone or even just with each other, I don't know how we would have gotten through it. Because even if you are Laurie Roth strong (and that's *really* strong!), you still have moments when cancer seems to be taking charge.

So we need people like you to come just at the right moment and whisper, "You will beat this. Cancer will not win." It is those few but perfect words that get us through another day. That's support. And when Laurie looked in the mirror and saw her head without her beautiful hair, it was you reminding her that she was as pretty as ever, and who needs hair anyway? That's support. And when we would wait for test results and the worry and anxiety in our hearts and minds could not be measured, you waited with us, you cried with us, and you have always rejoiced with us. That's support.

And when we offer up the annual women's basketball game honoring cancer survivors, on a cold Friday night in February, after everyone has had a very long week and all you want to do is go to bed or relax on your couch or do anything other than go back out, you come and you stand with us as beautiful Laurie triumphantly waves from midcourt, throwing kisses, and crying, knowing she has the very best family and friends a person could ever dream of. Now that's support.

You are the lights of our lives, and you make us better people just by being with us. "Thank you" doesn't seem like enough for people like you, but we'll say it anyway: thank you. From the bottom of our hearts, thank you. You are the absolute best.

Merry Christmas 2010
December 25, 2010

If you're receiving this email, then you have been a present that we were privileged to open before today. You are in our lives, blessing us, making us richer, making our lives better.

You have been with us on long, dark journeys. You have stood with us when cold winds blew a chill to the very marrow of our bones. You were with us when we had our own personal silent night. And here we are, celebrating life and hope and friendship, thanking God for another year of laughter and joys and good health. Let me rephrase that: GREAT health!

We found out a few years back that Christmas comes in different ways all through the year. From devastating news came perfect presents. They were wrapped beautifully in your love and support, faithfulness and friendship. You got us through, you held us close, and you helped make us believe that our midnight clear would come. In a few words, after long months of waiting, we knew the thrill of hope that allowed our weary world to begin rejoicing. Our silent night was over, our midnight clear had come, and we knew pure joy to our world.

We believed then what we believe now: our friends and family are our Christmas every single day of every year. You give us your best, you bring out our best. You fill our lives with love, you make our spirits bright.

To each of you and those you love, we wish you a Merry Christmas and a wonderful New Year.

Saying Goodbye to Max
April 28, 2011

It is with much heartache and sorrow that we tell you that we lost our little Maxie this morning. His life was far too short, his death came far too quickly, and our hearts will never be the same. Today, we struggle with just how fast this happened; tomorrow and all the other tomorrows, we will miss him in a way that words will never convey.

Max Jones was an original, and we were blessed to have his life cross ours. We lived with the court jester, the class clown, our very own Peter Pan. He was my sidekick, and I was his straight man, always marveling at his amazing personality. He brought smiles and laughs and sweet Maxie kisses to anyone he met. Life was to be lived in a hilarious way, and he made sure this house laughed a lot. To the very end, he truly never grew up, and we would have had it no other way.

I lost a piece of my soul today. Laurie lost her little man. Journey's main guy now watches from above. This one little boy filled every corner and inch of this home with his big personality. We are comforted to know that he and my mom, best pals here on earth, are together again. Without a doubt, heaven's newest angel is already working the crowd.

Dare to Be Different
September 14, 2011

In a sea of pink shirts, pink hats, pink shorts and shoes at this year's Race for the Cure, one team stood out. It was not because of their collective beauty or their true devotion to the one they walked in honor of, or even their deep love for me, your team captain. What set Laurie's Lifesavers apart was their unwavering willingness to follow one yellow noodle all over the race course. This commitment, this "eyes on the prize" attitude, this "daring to be different" character is what makes your captain proud!

It's easy to follow the crowd, to be like everyone else, to don our pink and off we go. It takes a special group to follow a yellow noodle and follow it proudly. I applaud you, Tina K., for the creative and courageous genius you displayed when you boldly strode through the pink crowd with your homemade yellow noodle shaped like a ribbon. (I also marvel that you didn't get beat to a pulp, but let's not dwell on that.) I tear up at the memory of your dramatic presentation to me, saying "Here—it's the best I could do in the time that I had," as you handed me the new team symbol for Laurie's Lifesavers. After all, yellow means joy and happiness—traits that each of the lifesavers embody. And yellow is the universal color for friendship. Nobody does friendship better than each of you! Is it any wonder, then, that a yellow noodle is our new mascot?

And beyond the outpouring of love and support on race day, Laurie's Lifesavers raised a record amount: $1,415! Wow! Big thanks to our donors and to those who walked with us in spirit! We always say that we do this for fun, but the funds that we raised will make an incredible difference to so many people in our community!

Laurie and I constantly thank our Lord for the friends that He has given us. It has been you who have gotten us through every leg of this long race. You have been racing for a cure for us since the day we heard the diagnosis. You have been our sunshine, our joy, and our happiness throughout this journey. You have reminded us that clouds are temporary, but hope is permanent. With hope, you can do a lot of things. With friends like you, we are completely unstoppable.

We could never thank you enough for all that you have done for us. The fact that you gave up the one Saturday that you got last week and walked beside us means the world to both of us. We know how busy life is, and yet you have never let it be too busy for us, no matter what we needed. May you always know that in our hearts and minds, you truly are our lifesavers.

From the bottom of my very humble captain (of the year) heart, thank you so very much for another awesome Race for the Cure!

PART 2
The Second Diagnosis

Breast Cancer Is Back
May 22, 2012

This is going to come as news to some of you, and I apologize for breaking it over email, but we received some tough news today. Unfortunately, Laurie has had a recurrence of her breast cancer. We are shell-shocked, devastated, and feeling a bit paralyzed with the news.

In a nutshell, we went for Laurie's routine mammogram last Thursday, where a concerning mass was found. After the ultrasound did not provide enough definition, she underwent a biopsy on Friday. We started the long wait at that point, and today we heard the news that we prayed we would not hear. The cancer is back, as is our fight.

The good news is that the mass is small (8 millimeters) and therefore, the eagle-eyed radiologist found it early. For that we are so very thankful.

Laurie will now undergo a full body scan (a PET scan), which we hope to have done as early as tomorrow or Thursday. We will then receive the results of that scan a few days later. As has always been par for our course, we will more than likely not receive the results until after this holiday weekend. That's okay—it gives all of us more time to think positively, visualize nothing but the good news that the cancer has not traveled outside of Laurie's breast, and send up prayers for her continued strength and peace.

Once we know about the scan, we will let all of you know. This road is familiar to all of us, isn't it? A road that we never wanted to take one single step on, and yet here we are. Here we are, with each of you beside us, each of you praying and holding us up with your love and support. As it has always been, our ace in the hole is Laurie. She's shocked now, but the fighter will soon come out, and when that fighter comes out—watch out, cancer. You thought she nailed you with her first punch? You have no idea how hard her second punch is!

This Is a Test, It Is Just a Test
May 24, 2012

Hello! Today is the day of Laurie's PET-CT scan. The PET scan is a full body scan that is capable of capturing images of changes in the body's metabolism caused by a growth of abnormal cells. The CT scan allows doctors to know the exact location of any changes.

Why are we doing this? Because we need to know if cancer has moved from Laurie's lump to anywhere else in her body. We pray that it hasn't. We are hopeful that this little 8-millimeter lump, undetectable by feel and able to be seen only with technology, stayed right there and didn't go anywhere else. Please pray this same prayer.

We will have the PET scan today and then meet with our oncologist, Dr. M., tomorrow for the results. It is the wait that is excruciating. You try to keep busy, you try to put your mind everywhere else, and yet no matter where you turn, there is the elephant in the room hogging all of your space.

God says if you have faith even the size of a mustard seed, you can move mountains. Most days, I think my faith is larger than a little ol' seed. Today the mustard seed may have me beat. Besides, moving mountains isn't my priority. Laurie is. All I want to do is move out of this nightmare as quickly as possible and give Laurie back the life she deserves—the life she fought so hard for four years ago.

Please pray and think positive thoughts for good results, continued strength, and faith, even as small as a little ol' mustard seed.

Not the News We Wanted
May 25, 2012

We are finally home from our appointment, and I wish I had better news of the results of the PET scan. Unfortunately, the clear results we were all shooting and praying for are not to be this time. The scan picked up areas that Dr. M. believes to be cancer. These areas are in her liver, a few spots on the lining of her right lung, and one spot on her spine. There are lymph nodes in the superclavicular area (right above the collarbone) that are also swollen. It was the laundry list we never wanted to hear recited.

Dr. M. actually went back to look at her scan himself because he was in disbelief. Her tumor markers from January were "perfect." And her energy level has been excellent. There are no other symptoms to point to these results. And yet here we sit.

Although Dr. M. has a treatment plan that he feels will work, he also suggested that we get a second opinion at Northwestern Memorial Hospital in Chicago. We are blessed to have the "experts of experts" in breast cancer just two and a half hours north of us. Sounds like a good plan to get them to take a look at Laurie and her scan and weigh in as to what they recommend.

Either way, chemo is in our future. There is a newer drug that will probably come into play for her, if Northwestern agrees. It will be combined with another tried and true winner to give cancer the one-two punch it so deserves. These chemo drugs are tough, but our Laurie is tougher. Cancer has forgotten who it's dealing with. We're about to remind it.

As you can well imagine, we are shocked beyond words. Our legs aren't of much purpose right now, and putting one foot in front of the other seems far too hard a job. Knowing Laurie, this paralysis won't last long. I will be forbidden to have pity parties, so I will have to do all of those on the sly. Laurie will get her feet under her, she will get her gloves on, and she will fight. She will fight like her life depends on it; she will fight because it does.

Laurie is a winner, she is a competitor, and most of all, she is a survivor. She will do this and she will win. Our Race for the Cure team is called Laurie's Lifesavers—and that's who you are. Together, all of us will cheer our champ on for the best victory lap ever taken.

Thank you for your continued prayers and all of your love. We are humbled by the love and support so deeply given to us. You truly are our lifesavers.

Wings Like Eagles
May 27, 2012

First, let us say thank you. From the bottom of our hearts, thank you for all the wonderful posts, for all the emails, the phone calls, the texts, and the visits. For each of you who has said a prayer, sent positive energy our way, thought of us throughout your busy day—thank you. We feel your love and are buoyed by your support. When our hearts go to the darkest of places, we find our minds taking us to you, to your thoughts, to your love. You're who we need, and you arrive right when we need you the most. Thank you.

These have been a tough couple of days (my new understatement of the year). In fact, we wake up and we pray that it was all a bad dream. We then remember that we are still in the midst of this nightmare. I look at Laurie and I know that she is in a state of disbelief, she is scared, she is hurting from the worry that comes with the words we heard on Friday afternoon. I feel my heart begin hurting to the point that it may be actually breaking in two. So I go directly into defensive mode, and God has heard some not-so-nice things from me.

I have flat-out said to Him, "Why her?" Since Laurie would never say it, I will and have. I remind God that she's had her turn in this awful barrel. This frightening road is very familiar territory in her not-so-distant past. So why not move along to someone else? I've been nice enough to point out people I see along the way and say, "Why not him?" "Why not her?" "Why not me?" To take this away from Laurie would be my dream come true right now.

I've even dared to think about uttering "How dare you?" but decide against pushing my luck with the Big Guy upstairs. And just when I was closing up one of my talks with Him, I was given a message of sorts. I was looking at Laurie and saw her actually laughing while playing with our dogs. Her face was filled with her beautiful smile, and her body looked lighter, not so heavily burdened with the words of last Friday. And I thought to myself how amazing she is—to be able to laugh and smile, to actually be up and moving, to be living right now when it would be so much easier to lie down.

And then I realized that this person will carry the message of hope and fight and determination better than anyone I had been pointing at, certainly better than me. When Laurie talks to you, you hear sweetness and kindness and not one ounce of bitterness. When Laurie smiles, you are enveloped in her absolute, unconditional love. And the way Laurie lives, it is a life of pure grace. I have said it before and I will say it again, she is grace under fire no matter the circumstances.

Does she want to muster up the fight that she knows all too well it will take to fight this beast? Not for one second. Will she? With every fiber of her body, yes, she will. Is she always smiling and laughing? Absolutely not, because her heart and mind are scared, rightfully so. Is she already facing this beast with hope and determination and perseverance? You'd better believe it. I am reminded of Isaiah 40:31, which says, "but those who hope in the Lord will renew their strength. They will soar on wings like eagles; they will run and not grow weary, they will walk and not be faint." Laurie is already beginning to soar; she's priming up for the fight; she is showing all of us, right now, right here, how to live.

Thank you, God, for making her with extra strength, extra resolve, extra fight. This gentle, easy spirit has a belly full of fire, and cancer is about to find out that it messed with the wrong person. And thankfully, we have an army of all of you behind us to do some reminding too.

We now await the date of the appointment with Northwestern. We need it to be soon so that they can weigh in on the right treatment plan and then get that started. Please pray that this happens in the time that we need it to.

You are our army of angels—each and every one of you. How blessed we are to have you in our lives. Thank you.

Angels Among Us
May 30, 2012

It's been a long couple of days as we anxiously awaited the phone call telling us whether we would be able to get into Northwestern's breast cancer center for a second opinion. God allowed me to practice not just my patience, but also my diplomacy, as I made a few (or twenty) follow-up phone calls and seemingly could not get this journey on the right path.

We had been told by Dr. M. that if we couldn't get into Northwestern within a week or two of last Friday, we would have to move forward without their opinion and start chemo. The aggressive timeline was in direct correlation to what could be an aggressive beast. So when we received a call from Dr. M.'s office saying that our appointment was June 15, a full three weeks from being given the PET scan results, we went into a bit of a tailspin. His nurse Katie quickly assured us that Dr. M. was okay with this wait. We made her reassure us three times, actually, and were not fully confident in the answer. After all, we don't need cancer to gain any more ground. But there was only so much Katie could do, and we needed to let it go. We needed to let it go and let God take hold of this. And boy, did He. He had this fully under control. He had a plan—He always does, and eventually I am going to learn that lesson.

He reminded us that we have many, many angels walking among us—each of you are counted on the angel list. We have a dear friend who is a nurse in Chicago who worked very hard today to get our appointment bumped up. Unfortunately, there was no movement due to the full schedules of this fabulous hospital. Thank you for trying and for all of your support, Lynne!

And we had another angel, my nephew's sister-in-law, Megan. She was a doctor at Northwestern not too long ago and still had many contacts there. When we first battled this in 2008, Megan was quick to offer to help us in any way she could. Her willingness to get involved continues, and this week was no exception. Not only did she get involved, she got us right to the top.

I have tears in my eyes as I type this and tell you that on June 6 at noon, Laurie and I are meeting with Dr. G. at Northwestern Hospital. Dr. G.'s name may not mean anything to you, but it means the world to me. I am the dork who for years has been reading anything by him that I can get my hands on. I am the nerd who wanted to go to one of his symposiums a few years back, but doing so would have required that I pose as a doctor and possibly be arrested as a stalker. Dr. G. is the doctor of doctors, and we will meet with him, he will have all of Laurie's information, and he will make the decision as to the best treatment for her. Praise the Lord!

I am deserving of a big "I told you so" from God, but thankfully, He doesn't work that way. Nor is He one bit surprised that I faltered, that I worried, that I went down to my knees. He knows His humble servant, and He knows this can be par for my course. But when I was on my knees, I looked up. I looked up, nodded to God, laid it all in His hands, and said, "Lord, this is all yours." Laurie's been special to God long before she was special to me. He has a plan for her, and He always will.

God had it in His hands all the while, working in the wings to make this happen just like it should. Thank you, God. Thank you, Megan, Megan's friends, and Dr. G. for being willing to fit us in. Thank you, Lynne, for making all your calls and trying all you could. Thank you to each and every one of you who said a prayer, sent out positive energy, and held us in your hearts over the past days. You are warriors, you are angels, you truly are Laurie's Lifesavers!

Time can't go fast enough!
June 4, 2012

This post is primarily to thank each and every member of our army who has called, posted, sent a card, stopped by, said a prayer, thought positively, sent an email, or shared our story with others.

Warning! Here comes an understatement alert: we are humbled by your love and support. Wow—how very blessed we are!

And the timing of each one is simply, and not surprisingly, divine intervention. When we are feeling anxious, your email reminds us to stay focused and trust in the path until we know the plan. When we feel so weary from this worry, you stop by and give us a hug and make us laugh and remind us that life is about all the minutes of the day, not just the ones that take our breath away. When we are feeling scared, your call comes in that encourages us to remember that we are not alone, that this fight will be fought with the power of God and all of you, our angels, not to mention the strongest person around, the invincible, amazing, and absolutely undefeatable Laurie Roth!

We head up to Northwestern on Wednesday, bright and early, for our appointment at noon with Dr. G. Frankly, Wednesday cannot come soon enough! Please pray that we are given the guidance and direction with which to fight this beast. We are anxious to get the treatment plan and get Laurie in the fight. My hope and prayer is that the wisdom of Dr. G. and the grace and guts of Laurie are the exact one-two punch that cancer needs to send it running for the hills!

We will post again when we get back. Until then, from the bottom of our humble hearts, thank you, our dear, sweet angels.

We like this opinion!
June 6, 2012

We have just gotten home from our trip to Northwestern and are feeling many emotions, all of which are good ones. We had an awesome consultation with Dr. G. and his nurse practitioner, Kelly. They spent a lot of time with us, gathering additional information, examining Laurie, and then sitting back down with us to recommend various treatment options. Yes, folks, I said *"various treatment options"*! While we would have been good with him just signing off on the treatment recommendation of Dr. M., the mere thought that we have "options" puts us over the moon!

The first thing that they made very clear was that if the spots on the PET scan are cancer that has metastasized to distant sites, they treat this as a chronic disease. Those words alone allowed both of us to begin breathing again. Chronic we can deal with.

They then said that they first want to have a biopsy of the spot on Laurie's liver. They are not optimistic that it is not cancer, since one of breast cancer's favorite places to travel is the liver, even though I've been highly recommending that it travel to the Bermuda Triangle. I've heard it's nice there for cancer this time of year. So it's likely that the spot on her liver is cancer. But breast cancer treatment, like that of many cancers, has become very specialized and very targeted. Rather than assume that the cancer in the liver has the exact same receptor and/or protein makeup as what we know is in Laurie's breast, we will use the biopsy to make that determination, and the treatment plan then will be extremely specific. Extremely specific, very targeted, the exact treatment it takes to knock cancer out of the park.

Since it seems pretty sure that it is cancer in the liver, we asked the doctor questions regarding the treatment. It was at this point that I felt my heart begin to move from the pit of my stomach back up to where it should be. Dr. G. began rattling off one chemo agent after another. He talked about fighting this beast with one agent, then said we could use another, then he talked about combining agents, and the list went on and on. He talked about oral chemo that Laurie could take in pill form once a day that have very few side effects. It was here that I began to see Laurie's face lift a little, and I assumed her heart was on an upward glide now too.

Always one to never take the wimpy way out, she asked if the oral chemo is as strong as chemo given in an IV. Dr. G. reassured us that it is equally strong and equally effective. There is just one area in which it isn't equal to chemo in a bag: the side effects. With the oral pill, Laurie gets to keep her hair, she shouldn't have mouth sores, and she shouldn't feel like she's been beaten by a hundred jackhammers. Nope, none of those. The side effects of the oral pill are few and sound pretty manageable. Amen to that!

In fact, we need a big ol' Amen to just about everything we heard today. We met with the best, he gave us options, and most of all, he gave us hope. When we were given this appointment with Dr. G., we knew God's plan was unfolding. I was reminded of God's word in Jeremiah 29:11, in which He says, "For I know the plans I have for you . . . plans to give you hope and a future." Today we got both. Today, with the multiple chemo options available and Dr. G.'s wisdom and reassuring manner, we were given hope. And trailing right beside hope was its very good partner, our future. Hope AND a future! Is there anything more beautiful?

And trailing right beside us, all the way to Chicago and back, was you. You, our army, our angels, our lights in the dark tunnel, the cheerleaders reminding us that this was the day that would bring the change our world needed to have. We left here with anxiety and panic sitting nervously in the backseat. (No, those are not nicknames for our dogs. Those, unfortunately, are two new emotions that set up camp a few weeks back.) We came home with relief and optimism proudly sitting front and center. You prayed for this day with us, you never took your eye off it, and you made us believe it could happen.

It not only could happen, it did happen. No matter what the biopsy shows, we have a plan. We've got Laurie with her new pink boxing gloves on and a boatload of chemo options ready if needed. We have faith in God and a trust in His plan. And we have you—we always have you, and that makes this plan the best ever.

Biopsy Is Set!
June 12, 2012

The word "biopsy" conjures up a simple needle stick, maybe two or three at the most. In reality, it can be a pretty serious procedure. The technicians could puncture a lung, they could knick a rib, or they could get needle happy and make a lot of sticks that could ultimately be quite painful for Laurie as she recovers. Yet when I called to tell her that we had a date and a time, her response was, "Oh, good. That will be great." Really? Considering I need sedation dentistry for a common cleaning, that would not have been my response to the same information.

But this is Laurie, the fighter, the warrior, the one with the new pink boxing gloves, and she is ready to start punching cancer out of her life. The biopsy starts the fight. It will be Laurie who ends the fight, and she will do so victoriously. But she knows that we need this information from the biopsy to guide the specific treatment from here on out. So she hears the news of another procedure, another test, another potentially painful weekend, and she says, "Oh, good. That will be great" and means every word of it.

When we get the results, we get on with the fight. When we get on with the fight, Laurie gets on with her life. Having seen her in this mode before, I have two words for cancer: WATCH OUT! It does not stand a chance. Not against Laurie, not against her army, not against all of you, Laurie's Lifesavers. It's the perfect combination knockout punch that will make cancer cower in the corner. I like that image, don't you?

Then, the following week, will see our oncologist, Dr. M., for the results. Still thankful for all the options Dr. G. rattled off last week, we will then all make the decision as to which option will work best. Whether it is chemo in a pill or chemo through her veins, it's still chemo, and we need to prepare for that and all the side effects it can bring. And yet, knowing our fighter the way that I do, when she hears the recommended option, Laurie will say, with all the grace and strength and courage that she always shows, "Oh, good. That will be great." Bless her heart. Bless her gutsy, ridiculously amazing, absolutely determined heart.

We will keep you up to date after the biopsy and again after we get the results. We are strengthened by your love, your comfort, your support. You are truly the brightest lights in our lives, a constant reflection of the love that God continues to shower down upon us. From the bottom of our grateful hearts, thank you.

Hurry Up and Wait!
June 15, 2012

I wanted to give everyone the update after the biopsy. Your girl did really well. And Laurie did well too.

As usual, our Laurie was a trouper. We arrived right on time, bright and early, at 7:00 a.m. The nurses got Laurie all prepped and ready to go and told us that it wouldn't be too long. Apparently, that's hospital speak for four hours. I'm not kidding.

But we tried to make the best of it. We read from the book *The Power*, which speaks of positive thinking and having good feelings and good emotions. The theory is that you get back what you have given out, whether positive or negative. By the sheer numbers of visits and posts to this site, your cards and emails and calls, it is clear that all the love that Laurie so effortlessly has sent out for so long is coming back tenfold. Thank you so much.

We whiled away the hours eavesdropping on other patients, listening to the nurses discuss their plans for the weekend, and convincing ourselves that many others have it much worse. We reminisced, we laughed, and we watched the clock. Just as I was about to launch into a musical number or the spellbinding recap of my family's vacation to California when I was seven, the tech came to get Laurie. Dang—I'll keep that story in my back pocket in case we need to burn up a couple hours again.

The biopsy itself took an hour. The radiologist was a pro and very capably got numerous tissue samples. This should give the pathologist a lot to work with to determine the makeup of the lesion. Amen.

Then the real fun started. The liver biopsy recovery process required that Laurie lie on her side for two hours to keep pressure on the wound site. That enjoyable position was then followed by an hour on her back—flat on her back, no elevation whatsoever. She was not able to be in any other position and certainly not able to stand up.

A liver biopsy also has some uncomfortable side effects: referred pain to the shoulder that starts out dull and then crescendos to a throbbing pain, pressure around the diaphragm, and certainly pain at the biopsy site. But despite all of that, our warrior took it all in stride, frequently refusing and not once accepting any pain medication. Her strength never ceases to amaze me. It was clear she was in pain, it was clear she was uncomfortable, but she chose to tough it out. As she explained to me, "I don't want to be knocked out for the rest of the day."

And there it is, folks. The attitude, the sheer determination, the constant focus that life is waiting for her and she's not missing a second of it. It's the guts-for-the-glory trade-off; it's making the choice to live, not lie down; it's the edge that she will always have on this beast. It will be, as they say, the difference maker. Thank you, Jesus!

Next up is our visit to Dr. M. on Monday afternoon for the biopsy results. That visit gives our champ the treatment plan, the type of chemo, the map for kicking cancer to the curb. Her boxing gloves are laced up and ready to go! This is when Laurie hits her stride—give her the plan, and out comes the fighter. Cancer will truly not know what hit it. I predict a TKO!

Thank you for being there beside us in the ring. Your strength, your support, your love is exactly the army we need surrounding us, holding us, cheering our champ on! You're the best. You're our army, and we love each of you with all of our hearts. Thank you so much.

It's Hammer Time!
June 18, 2012

We are home from our visit with Dr. M., our local oncologist. The liver biopsy did confirm that the growths in Laurie's liver are consistent with breast cancer. There is no reason to biopsy the spots on her lung or the one on her spine because the treatment plan would be the same regardless of their outcome. So since we know that breast cancer likes to go to the liver, lung, and bones, we will make the assumption that those are cancerous and knock those out with the proposed treatment plan.

Here is the plan: It will be a one-two punch of two chemo agents. One will be in pill form, called Xeloda (pronounced Zeloda), and one will be delivered intravenously, called Taxotere (pronounced "really mean drug that wipes out cancer"). Xeloda and Taxotere will be the cocktail specially made for Laurie (pronounced "bravest, most courageous person I know"). She will take the pill twice a day for fourteen days and then be off it for one week. She will receive Taxotere once every three weeks. Then, once a month she will receive a bone-strengthening drug that has anticancer properties, called Zometa. Zometa has made tremendous strides at not just building strong bones but knocking out bone cancer for breast cancer patients. Therefore, I pronounce Zometa our new best friend.

We've met Taxotere before. Laurie had that the first go-round, but it was combined with a totally different agent. What we know about it is that it could make her a little sick to her stomach, she probably will lose her hair, and it could make her tired. We also know that the last time she had it, she was never once nauseated (except that one time when I cooked, so I won't make that mistake again), she did lose her hair and looked absolutely beautiful, and she did more work than a crew of five guys throughout her treatment.

Xeloda and Zometa are new to us, but they get rave reviews from both Dr. G. and Dr. M. In fact, Dr. M. referred to Xeloda as a lethal hit to cancer cells. He said that Taxotere has always been one of the top winners. And he said that together, Xeloda and Taxotere are the hammer that we need to pound this beast into oblivion. Now, that's what I'm talking about!

For those of you old enough to remember (or unable to block out) the '80s video of MC Hammer dancing in his yellow harem pants, you will remember the constant refrain of "U can't touch this!" After giving us his recommendation, Dr. M. looked at us, smiled, and said, "It's hammer time." There was only one response, and we said it together: "U can't touch this!" Yes, admitting this makes me also admit that I'm humiliated for both of us. Yet it points to the incredible attitude of our champ. Faced with chemo, faced with side effects too numerous to count, faced with fear, she was able to laugh, to join the joke, and repeat one of the most ridiculous refrains ever sung: "U can't touch this!"

So, cancer, I say this to you: U can't touch her. You tried before, and you are trying again. But God made Laurie too strong to even bend for you, let alone fall down for you. Her indomitable spirit is too big, too mighty, too brave for little ol' you. Her determination has more force than any gale to ever blow through. And her faith and belief that she will win is beyond question. Get ready, cancer, our champ's gloves are laced, her dukes are up, her fight is on—it's hammer time!

Hammer time starts at noon this Thursday, when we sit down for the first chemo dosage of Taxotere. Please pray for Laurie's continued strength, both mental and physical. We feel all the love and positive energy you continue to pour onto us. We drink it up, and it brings us incredible comfort and renewed focus. You're our army of angels, our shining lights, our whispers of strength right when we need them the most. You truly are our lifesavers.

Did You Ever Know That You're My Hero?
June 21, 2012

If she didn't know it before, today cemented Laurie as my hero. I have a sneaking suspicion, though, that because I have mentioned it maybe once or one hundred times, she may have heard this before. If I hadn't spent the majority of the day threatening to go into the fetal position, I would have carried her on my shoulders.

We won't kid you—today was the day that started the fight we never wanted to get back into. It was the déjà vu moment that nobody wants to relive. Yet here we were, pulling into the cancer center with our bag of pictures, iPads, magazines, and all the items that get you through, walking up for chemo. It was the day we knew had to come, had to start, had to happen. It loomed in front of us like a freight train.

Laurie has a strength that is as much a part of her as the color of her eyes. It is innate; it is who she is; it is amazing. Her courage and bravery sometimes overwhelm me and, more often than not, move me to tears. She is truly grace under fire, weaving through painful tests and even more painful results, keeping her eye on the prize called life.

Today was no exception. Walking into the cancer center, I wanted to turn and flat-out run. I wanted to grab Laurie, toss her in the car, and keep driving. I stutter-stepped; I feigned like I had lost something in our bag; I went into a complete stall technique. Laurie? She walked straight to the door and walked bravely inside. This is the door that nobody wants to walk through. Behind this door are toxins, needles, and medicines that interrupt your beautiful life. This door rattles your bones, your nerves, your wonderful world. Through this door is where you go to get sick so that you can get better. And that, dear angels, is why Laurie so bravely walked through.

She walked through and sat down in the chemo chair, and we both knew it was hammer time. I had skipped wearing the parachute pants, thinking we had all suffered enough and did not need to deal with that sight. Instead, Laurie and I visualized positive things: each of you, Journey, Max, Harbour, and Alicat. We thought of beautiful memories made and the ones we plan to make in the future—the future that can't come soon enough.

"For I know the plans I have for you . . . plans to give you hope and a future." That's why Laurie walks through the door today and all the days she will have to. She has hope and she has a future, and those make all the difference in this fight. She knows that God is designing a future for her, and she is anxious to get it started. And God knows what I have always known: this world is a better, sweeter place with Laurie Roth in it.

So we're one chemo down. In the next couple of days we'll know how it will make Laurie feel. But we already know this: We have a bright, new, shiny pink hammer to beat cancer into submission. We have pretty pink boxing gloves with which the champ will remind cancer that "U can't touch this!" And we have you, the army of the very best friends and family two people have ever been blessed to share their lives with. We are truly humbled, warmed, and oh so grateful for each and every one of you, our wonderful, beautiful angels.

We will keep you posted on how our girl does. My bet is that she has a huge project waiting for us this weekend. Yikes! I am really going to have to buck up to keep up!

Did Anyone Catch the License on That Truck?
June 24, 2012

Well, I didn't quite catch the license plate on the truck that rolled over Laurie, but my guess is it read TAXOTERE. Our girl has had a rough couple of days as the medicine surges through her veins, fighting like mad to find those nasty cancer cells. Taxotere took "hammer time" to an all new meaning! Ironically, though, it's the cure, not the cancer, that is kicking butt and taking names. Unfortunately, one of those names it took is our Laurie's.

We're getting an in-your-face reminder of our old friend Taxotere. It is a mighty weapon in our fight, but it takes the good with the bad and leaves a destructive trail in its wake—a trail littered with mouth sores, depleted taste buds, fatigue, and body aches. "The flu times a thousand" is how we used to describe it, and that phrase is as apropos now as it was four years ago.

But the difference maker then is exactly the same as the difference maker now: it's Laurie. She wakes up with a headache, the kind that makes your eyes squint and each step more painful than the last. My response would be to get back in bed—bed always seems so reasonable. Laurie's response: "I'll feel better once I'm up and around." She has body aches that give her chills and hot flashes all at the same time. My response: "Hi, bed." Laurie's response: "These will pass." She has fatigue that makes a shower seem like a marathon, she has mouth sores and painful joints, and the list goes on and on. I think you know my response: "Just going to take a little snoozy." Laurie's: "I'll sit, but not for long."

She gets up, she showers, she dresses, and she lives. She remembers our refrain and wants to show cancer that "U can't touch this." Can't hit a moving target, right? She is always in fighter mode, folks. Always! And this fight will be won, because we have the champion fighter in the ring. Amen.

Right now, Taxotere is doing a lot of the heavy lifting, and Laurie is along for the not-so-fun ride. She's sure not giving in, but her body is being beat up by the cure. By tomorrow, if our notes from last time prove true, Laurie will begin to hit her stride. It won't be 100 percent better, but it will be a bit better. A bit better is what we're shooting for. Tomorrow can't come soon enough.

Please know that as we pass the time, we enjoy your posts, your emails, your cards, and your calls. Your spirit invades both of us, and we feel the strength of this magnificent army of family and friends. We're abundantly blessed by each of you. Thank you.

I'll be back in touch so you know how the champ is doing. I hear her out in the kitchen as I type. She's probably considering repainting it when she feels just a little bit stronger—I'm not kidding. But as I have that thought, I have this one: Thank you, Jesus, for making her so very determined, so very brave, so very strong. She will always be the difference maker—in this fight, in my life, in this world. Again, I say AMEN.

Calling All White Blood Cells!
June 28, 2012

This entry starts out like most of the others, with a heartfelt thank-you to you, our beautiful army of friends and family. Your support has been overwhelming, amazing, and so very appreciated. Every day, in some way, one or two or ten of you reach out, share your love, and remind us that we are not alone. You are the perfect lights guiding us through what can sometimes be a very dark storm. Who am I kidding? Storm? This is a Category 5 hurricane, and technically, we should be boarding up the windows and hunkering in the basement! But with you by our sides, we know our burden is shared, supported, and prayed for every day. The comfort you bring is the best medicine of all.

Speaking of medicine, we are one week out from the teaming up of Laurie, Xeloda, and Taxotere. Or as I like to refer to this trio, the Good, the Bad, and the Ugly. And man oh man, is Taxotere an ugly one. In its quest to obliterate the cancer, it races through Laurie's system searching for the enemy cells and wiping out everything in its wake. It's nondiscriminatory, taking the good cells with the bad ones. Taxotere is a bull in a china shop, and right now, we have a lot of cleanup before Laurie is back in business.

Today we saw Dr. M. Laurie's blood tests showed that the very important white blood cells were basically wiped out completely. Understatement alert: that's not good. In fact, that's really bad. It is a huge contributor to her fatigue, her headaches, her body aches. And yet our champ, with virtually no white blood cells in her entire system, had her best day yesterday. She walked the dogs, she walked the neighbor's dog, she cleaned the house, she even vacuumed. That last one may not sound overly impressive, but trust me, it is. Using our vacuum is the equivalent of pushing a Volkswagen around the house. I'm not kidding. It's that heavy. When I vacuum, I use both arms and both legs, usually have at least one of the dogs helping, and I'm still crawling around and straining behind it. Very often, I am whining. Bare bones minimum, I am audibly complaining the entire time. Laurie? She whipped it around the house like it was a feather duster. She always does, and yesterday was no exception.

Where does her strength come from? It's superhuman. She does what she has to do. She sucks it up, because any other option simply isn't one. The Bible tells us that God "gives strength to the weary and increases the power of the weak" (Isaiah 40:29). With her low level of white blood cells, Laurie should have been folded up and tucked under the sheets. She should have been both weak and weary. Instead, God whispered that she was not alone, that her army was behind her, and He was beside her, all the while increasing her strength. Amen.

Today she received a white blood cell booster shot. The shot was a must-have, because a count this low is very dangerous. She is ripe for infection, her fatigue has already gotten worse, and the headaches and bone aches are back in full swing. Some of those are actually the side effects from the shot. Once again, the very medicine that is curing her is knocking her around in its own way. Please pray that the booster takes effect quickly and our girl is up and vacuuming again very soon.

Two other areas that have been a challenge are food and her taste buds. Things taste like "salt licks" or very metallic. Through trial and error, we have found a few soups that Laurie can tolerate. She is basically existing on baked potatoes, yogurt, and smoothies. We'll probably add some Ensures or Boosts today, just to make sure that she's getting her nutrients. She tries hard to make this food thing work. But the grim reality is that most foods, all breads, and many liquids are, in a word, awful. Bless her heart, Laurie tries anything I put in front of her. She's secure in the fact that I didn't cook it and always optimistic that maybe, just maybe, it might not taste awful. We're no longer shooting for food to taste good. We just want it to not taste awful.

As always, no matter what she's facing, Laurie's beautiful spirit shines through. She gets up every morning, admittedly nervous about what side effects may rear their ugly heads, but she's still eager to start her day. She gets moving, even though bones ache and her head hurts, but there's a life to be lived and she's not missing out. She laughs during our appointments with Dr. M., because he is funny and we have always all cracked up with each other. I marvel that as weak as she is, as sick as she feels, as hard as her life is right now, she still laughs. It's a good, fun, Laurie Roth laugh, and it is always music to my ears.

She smiles at the people in the waiting room at the cancer center, then worries about them after we leave. She has actually said to me on numerous occasions, "Things could be so much worse. All

I need to do is look around." There's God increasing her strength again—helping her see life from someone else's perspective. She won't feel sorry for herself; there will be no "save the date" cards for an upcoming pity party; this will never, ever be all about her. Try as I might to help her see it that way, she reminds me that there are others worse off all around us. It is then, always then, that I look at her in complete amazement, try to hide the tears, and softly whisper, "Thank you, Jesus."

Here's the deal about Laurie: she does not see herself as sick. She won't ever see herself that way. She knows cancer is inside her, but she's fighting it with everything she's got. She's in it to win it, folks. She bobs, she weaves, she punches hard, she's moving fast and moving well. We told you, cancer, U can't touch her! She's the champ, the number one girl, the queen to this court jester. If she won't see herself as sick, far be it from me to do so. Yet today, seeing her right now, so wiped and so tired, that's a tall order.

Where Are You, White Blood Cells?
June 29, 2012

Our champ was knocked around and almost down a couple of times today. While we tried to get the white blood cell booster in her quickly, she probably already had the makings of some infection in her body. Early this morning she awoke to a pretty bad pain in her throat and a terrible headache. We knew exactly what was going on: infection. And without white blood cells, this could get dangerous in a heartbeat.

I called and spoke to Dr. M.'s nurse, Katie. She knows my voice before I say my name (she and Sara tolerate me really well), and immediately said, "How's our Laurie?" I told her the symptoms, and she confirmed what we already feared—this is an infection, and we have to get it under control immediately. So a high-powered antibiotic was called in. Laurie has had that going through her today and will stay on it for the next five days.

Remember when I mentioned that our old friend Taxotere causes side effects that are like the flu times a thousand? Well, the booster shot only adds to those wiped-out, painful side effects, at least for the first forty-eight hours as it moves to build up Laurie's immune system. This infection is the last thing that we needed, but not one bit surprising. It's part and parcel of the fight, par for the course, and familiar territory from the last time.

Cancer is never a fair fighter. Not only is cancer a meanie, but the very medicine that works to cure you can nearly knock you out of the game. The medicinal partners on your side of the rope can make you feel like they are actually working against you. They fight with such might that they take the good with the bad and leave you on your knees. They say only the strong survive—and thankfully, that's exactly who we have fighting this beast: the strongest person I know, Laurie Roth.

We all, myself included, need to remember that we had these same setbacks the last time, and our girl came shining through. She took the sucker punches of cancer and the cure and came out the victor. She got up when so many would have called "time out," would have slapped the mat, game over. Certainly I would have. Not Laurie. She stood up, she stared cancer down, and she lived to tell about it. That's what I'm talking about. That's *who* I'm talking about. That is our girl.

God is the great physician. He is holding Laurie as I type, as we pray, as she sleeps. Please pray for healing throughout her entire body. Please pray that all the medicine does what it needs to do—heal her aches, heal her infection, kill her cancer.

She needs a good day. Right now, we'd take even one. One would do the trick. Here's the deal: our girl has the patience of Job for 99.5 percent of life (a particularly handy attribute for dealing with this little ol' sidekick all these years), but not when it comes to not feeling well. I've always referred to her as my "impatient patient." She is here to live, not to lie around. She is here to make life better for others, not to rest on her laurels. She is here to make this world, my world, about as good as it gets. Every day that she's in it, she succeeds. May she always receive even nearly as much good as she gives.

Thank you, beautiful, wonderful angels. What would we ever do without you? Each and every one of you is a blessing in our lives.

Can I Get an Amen?
June 30, 2012

Nicely done, army of friends and family! While our girl isn't 100 percent, maybe not really even 50 percent, she's better than she was when I wrote last night. Actually, she's better than she was throughout the night and early this morning. Scary times then, better times now. Whew.

Her headache is better, her body aches are better, and her throat infection seems to be moving in the right direction. God hears all of our prayers, and it is abundantly clear that He answered the prayers of His faithful people last night and early this morning. AMEN! Bless Laurie's beautiful heart—she'll take 50 percent and run with it. I just hope I can keep up!

She's still susceptible to infection, so we have to be vigilant about that aspect. She feels a little like the boy in the bubble. I feel like her bodyguard. I am an obsessive-compulsive hand washer, so keeping things clean and disinfected is a breeze. However, trying to keep Laurie confined is no easy feat. God brought the oppressive heat to help my cause and keep her inside. If things continue on an upswing today, we'll get out for a bit, maybe a drive, maybe to the lake. These four walls were never meant to hold Laurie. And again I say, "Thank you, Jesus."

So a big thank-you to all of you for your prayers, your positive thoughts, your love, and your support. Let's keep those going and pray that Laurie continues on this upward glide. You're an amazing army of angels taking care of one of God's best. From her thankful heart and my humbled one, thank you so much.

To All Our Yankee Doodle Dandies!
July 4, 2012

Just a quick update before all of us start our Fourth of July celebrations. We're at midweek, but it seems like light-years from where we were just five short days ago, when Laurie was so very sick. We reached out to you, you reached up to heaven, and God put His healing hand on her and carried us through a very scary couple of days. We continue to be thankful for the wonderful and amazing healing that has taken place.

Throughout this week, your funny, sweet, oh-so-thoughtful cards, emails, posts, and calls have poured in, sending your love right to our hearts. We savor the support, relishing the blessings and love that each one of you sends to us and finding renewed strength right when we need it most. You come to us through this site, through the mail, in person, and in spirit. We are sometimes overwhelmed, yet always appreciative of the love each one of you showers upon us. Thank you.

This has been a better week in terms of pain and discomfort, allowing Laurie to find a new normal. Not the one she wants or would ever choose, but one that allows her to enjoy the day, take the dogs swimming, and yes, even vacuum. While this journey will never be a walk in the park by any stretch, Laurie faces the side effects with her usual grace, her constant courage, and her determined focus that this beast will be beaten down, beaten up, beaten out. I see her pushing through, knowing full well that I would fold like a house of cards, and yet she stands tall. I sit (I could end the sentence right there) in constant awe of her ability to put mind over matter, to find the strength to dig deep and past the pain to fight the beast. To her, there is no other choice. This is a fight that Laurie's life depends on, so our girl will settle for nothing less than a TKO. Amen!

So on this Independence Day, while we would love to have freedom from so many things that have arrived over the past six weeks, we accept that chemo, body aches, taste changes, and the flu times a thousand are all part of the process, part of the team, part of the fight. We get that Taxotere, Xeloda, and low white blood cell counts are going to have to knock Laurie to her knees on some days so that she can soon stand victorious on all her days to come. I have to constantly remind myself that Laurie, the most gentle spirit I have known, can't have independence from any of this right now. She has to endure the pain, team up with the poison, find the fire in her belly every second of every day so she can live freely, live fully, and in one simple, beautiful word, live.

However, what we would never, ever want to be is independent of all of you. Today and every day, you truly are our Yankee Doodle

Dandies, strengthening us and comforting us, loving us through it every step of the way. While I already live in the home of the brave, I know that through your love, God's love, and the fighter that is Laurie, we will all soon live in the land of the free. Free of worry, free of pain, free of cancer. And that, dear Dandies, will be our new Independence Day!

As Beautiful Today as Every Other Day
July 9, 2012

I wanted to give you all an update on our girl. This has been a pretty darn good group of days. And that's the cruel joke of chemo. Just as you are beginning to taste again, just as your body feels only a little flu-like and not a lot flu-like, just when the headaches begin to go away, it's time to go in for another dose. Clearly, chemo is not known for its comedic tendencies, because that one really falls flat. But you know our champ—she's grateful for the good days and knows that the bad ones, while not one bit fun, are all part of the process. She truly takes the good with the bad.

This was the time frame, however, that brought about the ever-dreaded day fourteen. Day fourteen is the day that we knew was coming; in fact, we'd had it on the calendar since the first day Taxotere went racing through Laurie's veins. Day fourteen is the day that comes whether you want it to or not, and when it leaves, it has taken your hair with it. Even as day fourteen turned into evening, and Laurie dared to hope that maybe, just maybe, she had dodged a bullet, her hair was falling out. Even as I teared up at this additional thing that she had to endure and had hoped might not happen, it was happening. Even as she bravely went and picked up her favorite hat to ready herself for what would happen, her hair was trailing her. So many times I have made Laurie want to pull her hair out, but this time, Taxotere made it all too easy.

There are few things so devastating to people as when they lose their hair to chemo. And if you know Laurie, then you know that there is rarely, if ever, a hair out of place. Her hair is really pretty, it's spunky, it's fun. In a word, it's Laurie. So just when we were on the upward glide, just when the new normal was feeling almost like the old normal, just when Laurie was feeling like herself again, she looked in the mirror and didn't know who was looking back at her.

Personally, having seen Laurie go through this and lose her hair, I know that Laurie is as beautiful on day fifteen and day sixteen as she ever was on day eleven or day seven or the day when we didn't even know this journey was going to come our way. God gave her a beautiful face, with high cheekbones and almond-shaped eyes and the cutest darn egg-shaped head that He ever created. In fact, kudos to God on that head—it is perfect! Unlike mine . . . I'm serious. Laurie will back me up on that, as she did when I feebly offered to shave my head too. She did not even attempt to hide her look of horror as she yelled "NO!" She then got a grip, punched it up a bit, and said, "Oh, gosh, that's so sweet, but so not necessary." Talk about dodging a bullet! Proving that I am often found on the low road, I breathed a big ol' sigh of relief, and every single one of you should do the same.

Let me tell you about day fifteen and day sixteen: Our champ was sporting cute caps, looking great, feeling better, and walking through the crowd with her usual grace and beautiful spirit. God didn't just make a perfectly shaped head, He made such a brave soul who keeps showing us that life has to be lived in rain clouds the same as we live it in the sunshine. Amen.

As a self-proclaimed cockeyed optimist (insert: not really grounded in reality), I don't like thinking of it as her hair "falling out." That seems too negative. Instead, I'm reminded of one of my favorite children's books, *The Velveteen Rabbit*. Don't ever ask my sister about it, because she can quote most of it, and that is just as annoying as it sounds. Anyway, if you don't know the story, in a nutshell, it's the magical tale of how our beloved toys in our toy boxes become "real." The quote that I love takes place in a conversation between the Skin Horse and the Velveteen Rabbit. The Skin Horse has been around in the toy box for many years, and the Velveteen Rabbit is new to the nursery. The Velveteen Rabbit wants to become as real as the Skin Horse and asks him how best to go about this. The Skin Horse, who has a tattered brown coat with seams that have been rubbed off by the little hands of the children who have lovingly held him as they slept, as they cried, as they lived, explains gently to the Velveteen Rabbit, "Generally, by the time you are Real, most of your hair has been loved off."

That's how I see Laurie right now. Her hair has been loved off. I no longer see it as "fallen out," taken by Taxotere, gone thanks to chemo. Nope. It's been loved off. Loved off by you, by our families, by me; by God, who not only created that head but knows every hair He put in it; by every angel in our life who we don't even know but who prays for us every single day. She's as real as they get, the best of the best, and we love the heck out of her. We love her with hair or without, we love her to the moon and back, we love her always and forever. And when we celebrate the TKO, we will love her hair right back on again.

So as we go through this week, we do ask for your prayers. We need prayers for Laurie's continued strength, continued willpower, continued health. In fact, right now I am a little concerned about a tightness Laurie has in her chest and am worried that it could be the sign of an infection. Back on the antibiotic we go, so that our champ is fit as a fiddle to fight the beast. Please pray that the antibiotic works its magic like it did the last time.

Thank you to each one of you, our beautiful army of angels and lifesavers. How blessed we are to have you in our lives.

Grateful Hearts
July 12, 2012

We decided to take a different tack this time as we went into the chemo ring. Instead of me moving into the fetal position (not your best fighting position, even for a wingman) and instead of Laurie faking that this was really no big deal, we decided to approach it from another angle. While we will probably never be the ones "grateful to have cancer," we decided that despite this diagnosis, we are surrounded by so much for which to be thankful. We decided to take stock of that, thank God for our blessings, and move forward from there.

Of course, at the top of our list is each one of you. Greater blessings, greater gifts, have never been given. You are the cheerleaders on this marathon, the angels whispering words of support and love, the tag-team fighters ready to beat cancer silly when Laurie needs to put the gloves down for a bit and rest. This is a journey taken one step at a time, and even one baby step can feel like a tall, tall order. Yet with you beside us, we are strengthened, we are supported, we are loved. Bless each one of you for all that you give to us each and every day, each and every step of the way.

We also prayed gratefully for the amazing team of the talented Dr. M., his wonderful nurses, and the arsenal of medicines that we have just two blocks from our house. We so appreciate that all the resources to beat this beast are right down the road from where we live. Personally, my heart overflows with thankfulness for the person God made in Laurie Roth: stronger than average, sweet to the inner corners of her beautiful soul, and determined to never, ever lose. She is a winning combination of grit and guts and grace. She is my own personal superhero with whom I am privileged to share my life. I truly believe that with the right amount of white blood cells, she could leap tall buildings in a single bound!

Speaking of white blood cells, they decided to stick around this time. Laurie had a whopping 8.6 white blood cell count—an all-time high for our girl! Little show-off! Of course, we know that the Taxotere and Xeloda will cause the cells to tank, which then leaves Laurie very vulnerable to all things germy. So to get ahead of this a bit, Laurie will have a booster shot tomorrow to begin building these important little guys right back up. We are grateful that Dr. M. chose a proactive route to give Laurie the best chance at staying healthy while the chemo does its job.

And when we look around the cancer center and see the people fighting for their lives, we are thankful that *this* is the journey God gave us. As Laurie often says, it could be so much worse. I used to debate her a bit on that, working to convince her that this *is* a bad one—that this is our "worse," and therefore, it has to be the very worst. Laurie would never buy it, not for a minute, quickly reminding me that so many have it so much worse. On our very first time back in the chemo room for this fight, as I tearfully took a look around, she made me a believer in her selfless, amazing mantra. Oh Lord, she was right. It could be so much worse. Thank you, God, for enabling Laurie to help me see the silver lining, the sunshine, the rainbow in between these very dark clouds.

So our fighter has her big guns running through her: Taxotere, Xeloda, and Zometa. They are fighters of the toughest kind, joining forces with the consummate fighter of them all: Laurie. She will feel beat up by their zest to find every single cancer cell, and on those days, she'll need to take it easy. If this round is like the last one, she'll hit her stride about seven days in and begin to feel a little better, a little stronger, a little more like Laurie Roth. She'll start making her lists of landscape projects and household must-dos, and our daily runs to Menards and Lowe's will resume. She will laugh and make me laugh with her; she will smile, and even if it's at night, anyone around will think the sun came out; and she will gracefully walk around brightening this world, my world, like nobody else ever has. And for that, I will be forever grateful.

The Healing Power of Pets
July 17, 2012

We have just arrived back home from our follow-up appointment with Dr. M. The routine is that Laurie gets chemo, and then five to seven days later we get her blood checked, meet with Dr. M., and tell him the side effects. Today's report was very good—all of her blood work looks good to him, even the pesky white blood cells that keep disappearing. Laurie's had dropped a bit, but Dr. M. still thought that they were in a good range. We'll take that!

Her side effects have been a little different this time. The good news is that the fatigue has not been as bad. We've weathered this one without a headache. But she has had mouth sores and tongue sores, making eating and talking difficult. Those continue to impact her taste buds, so nothing tastes right, very little tastes good, and we still strive to have things "not taste awful." "Not awful" is a good thing. Who knew? We've tried a homemade mouth rinse that helped a bit, but we are now getting a prescription concoction to hopefully get this side effect a bit more under control.

Another new side effect that appeared this round is very painful fingernails. Laurie said it feels like each finger and each thumb has been hit a dozen times by a hammer. This was not the hammer time we had in mind!

The fact of the matter is that with Taxotere, Laurie's fingernails could actually fall out—do you believe that? Thank goodness chemo kills cancer, because it would not be invited anywhere with the way it behaves! The pain she is experiencing just from the pressure under each nail is bad enough. I cannot even imagine Laurie having to deal with them falling out. I pray every day that enough is enough and that her fingernails stay right where they are. Please pray this with me.

And yet, even though opening a jar or turning the car key or anything that puts the least amount of pressure on her nail will cause her to grimace, one thing always makes her smile: petting our dogs, Journey and Harbour. They are fabulous nurses and never fail to make our spirits bright. They sit by Laurie when she has actually agreed to rest; they walk with her when she goes through the yard checking each flower like the baby that it is to her; they look at her with deep brown eyes, and those eyes shower her with pure love. It is a medicine that, if bottled, would be worth millions. These days, in our lives, it is priceless.

As many of you know, Laurie runs a pet therapy program through which a group of us bring our dogs to area nursing homes. It was a program started about twenty-five years ago by our dear friend Linda C. She had this marvelous idea to bring people and pets together to promote wellness. In fact, she named the group PAW to PAW, with PAW being an acronym for "people, animals, and wellness." Laurie and I have always found that if we have the first two, we usually get the third. When we have our pets, our lives are well. Even when our lives aren't so well, they certainly make it so much better.

This week we've temporarily added another pet to the tribe. He's a one-and-a-half-year-old golden retriever named Duke. He's actually Journey and Harbour's nephew, and they never let him forget it! Duke's family is on vacation, and we were fortunate enough to get to watch this fifty-five-pound bundle of hilarity. His family worried so much that this was not good timing and that they should make other arrangements. We insisted that Duke still come, knowing that he was going to be just what we needed right now. He has made us laugh very hard every single day, generally more than once. Life is funny to Duke, and watching it through his eyes makes it funny to us.

The irony is not lost on me as I watch Laurie with all of our pets and the amazing healing powers they give to her. This person who has devoted years and years to taking her pets to people, hoping to bring them a smile, maybe a laugh, but always a lot of love, is now getting that love back tenfold from our two dogs, from Mr. Duke, and even from our cat, Ali. I say "even Ali" because Ali does not give love, she takes it. She takes it on her own terms and her own time, usually at 2:30 in the morning, when she knows she is waking you and disturbing you the most. Right now, Ali is clearly making an exception for Laurie–although I've cautioned Laurie not to get used to it. Ali can turn on a dime, easily making the fingernail-falling-out thing look like a day at the spa!

So between all your love and our pets' love, you've made this beautiful Laurie sandwich. She's squished on one side by your calls and cards, your prayers and positive thoughts. And on the other side, our pets slather her with kisses too many to count, gentle spirits letting her know that they are always with her, and deep brown eyes that seep deep into her soul and bring incredible comfort. Now that's a recipe to be repeated! I'd order a Laurie sandwich any day!

We have our next chemo on August 2, but I'll be in touch before that so that you know how our girl is doing. We will have the next PET scan in mid-August to see how well Taxotere and Xeloda are pummeling cancer. We hope and pray that cancer is cowering, whining, packing its bags, and running to the nearest door. We hope and pray that it is leaving the building, exiting stage left—adios, sayonara, goodbye to you, cancer. We hope and pray that after all that Laurie has endured, she will be given her life back. My daily prayer is "Please, Lord, let that be the news."

Thank you for all that you do and are to us. We are the luckiest people to share our lives with you.

Taking the Good with the Not So Good
July 24, 2012

So if there is one thing this journey definitely teaches, it's patience. Patience through the tough times, patience through the pain, and patience through really awful side effects. Because once you learn patience, you move on to hope. And when you have hope, you hold the ticket that lets you see the day that we know is coming—the day when Laurie stands victorious in the ring, arms held high, cancer nowhere in sight, and all of us cheering for our champ as loudly as this great group can yell.

That's the day I try to keep in the forefront of my mind as I watch Laurie muscle through the not-so-good days. Unfortunately, this was a week and weekend that brought the good with the bad. She felt pretty good, or as good as a person can feel who is taking two different and extremely strong chemo drugs. She managed to work in a project or two that I had absolutely no desire to tackle. But how do I wimp out when the person with chemo running through her veins is lining up the tools? She managed to get some things crossed off the ol' to-do list that have been nagging at her. She managed to do a lot of things because, as far as she was concerned, she felt pretty good. Laurie Roth can do more on "pretty good" than a construction crew can accomplish.

She grabs for the gusto when she feels good. Let me tell you, she grabs it and she runs with it. And as much as I tease her (and whine all the while I'm helping), I love every second of it. Because the whole time she is checking off items on her list—laying new brick by the patio (I'm not kidding) or doing whatever it is that pops into her head that has to get done—she's winning. She's showing cancer that no matter what it tries to do to her, she will keep swinging, keep fighting, keep living. I have said it one thousand times: cancer messed with the wrong person!

And it is this same Laurie Roth who, when the cure knocks her down, makes her joints throb, and makes her skin hurt, will for the most part say to me, "It's working to make me better." Who says that? She takes the good with the bad; she appreciates the days when she can work around the house, play with the dogs, laugh with *and* at me. She knows those are great days and gifts that she has been given. But she is real enough to know that the not-so-good days will also be part of this journey. The grim reality is that she has to feel worse to feel better. While she may not like that, she knows that's how this fight is won.

This weekend was a roller coaster ride, and Sybil was at the controls. One day was good and one day was terrible. And when terrible hits, it hits with a vengeance. It hit so hard, it scared me. Scared me so much that I suggested that Laurie not take the oral chemo. I was that desperate for her poor body to be given some sort of break. As strong as Laurie is, I know we humans are all made with a breaking point. Mine comes early and often, without one ounce of shame, and usually with me announcing it. To date, Laurie's breaking point has yet to even show up. No matter what I've seen her deal with, I've never seen a breaking point. Yet Sunday night, as sick as she was, as bad as she felt, as weak as she could be, I thought for the first time since I met her, she might just be at her breaking point.

As soon as I suggested taking a break from Xeloda, it was like God whispered into her ear and reminded her of how He designed her. In Laurie Roth, God did not make a wimp. Inside her He tucked Herculean strength, legs to go the distance, and a determined focus to never take her eyes off the prize. When she seems to be on the ropes, Laurie digs deep down and pulls out sheer determination so that she can do nothing other than win. So when I suggested backing off, Laurie looked at me and said, "I have to take it. I have to fight. I want this next scan to look as good as it possibly can." As I sat by her, tears streaming down my face, I whispered a very humble, very appreciative, and very relieved "Amen."

Today is better. Today she found lots of things to do to keep busy, to keep fighting. After her yesterday and her Sunday night, I'm not sure how she does it. Is it willpower? Is it that superhero coming out in her? Is it that this is just one of the good days? I think it is all of the above. But whatever the reason, the good day is here, we're going to take it, and we're going to enjoy it.

We did find out today that Laurie's next scan will be on Monday, August 13. This is the scan to see how things are looking inside her. Let's pray that these powerful toxins that are ripping her body apart are also ripping cancer into tiny, soon-to-be-nonexistent shreds. Let's pray that she is able to endure her next chemo on August 2 with as few of these nasty side effects as possible. And let's pray that our champ is soon standing victorious in the ring, arms over her head, and all of us cheering her total knockout of this beast called cancer.

I'm wrapping this up now. I hear the chain saw firing up to cut tree limbs for tomorrow's garbage day—again, I'm not kidding, and I'm absolutely loving it!

This Is Livin'!
August 1, 2012

So here we are on the eve of Laurie's third chemo treatment, and she's feeling pretty well. So well, in fact, that many people in her place would consider not going for the treatment. Of course, our champ knows she must have the chemo, despite knowing what comes of it.

The first week of chemo is awful, as you well know from what we have shared: the pain, the infections, the near total tsunami that washes over Laurie, taking so much in its wake. Her climb out of that calamity begins sometime in the second week. It's during the second week that she begins to trim trees, add on to patios, and power wash the windows. She is energized not so much by actually feeling better, because she barely does, but rather by showing cancer who is in charge. Cancer may bend her, but it will not break her. So just to drive the point straight into cancer's face, Laurie fires up the chain saw.

The third week is when Laurie hits her stride. It's not pain-free, but it's an improvement, and she's grabbing for every ounce of life she can find. It is her week and hers alone. She smiles more, she laughs more, she *lives* more. This is the week that she has earned after dealing with mouth sores and finger pain and stomachaches. This is the week when she visits with friends, when she fishes and reels in the big ones in the lake, when we go out to eat and she actually enjoys the food that we paid for. This is the week when we sit on the deck, look at each other, and say our favorite old refrain: "This is livin'!"

This really is livin', because this is the week that reminds us of what we are shooting for. Our new normal begins to remind us of our old normal. Not to brag, but our old normal was pretty darn good—so very blessed, so much fun. We have great families, great friends, and Journey, Harbour, and Alicat always willing to entertain. Well, Ali is always willing to bite, but Journey and Harbour are Laurel and Hardy. So much so that after watching their antics, we often wonder why we pay for cable. This is the week when we go out to dinner, me ordering steak, Laurie ordering halibut (just for the halibut—sorry, couldn't resist). We sit there, seemingly without a care in the world, enjoying our life. This is the week we find our old life and savor every minute of it!

I credit Laurie for helping us have this week. Her master plan is that life will be as normal as possible. With pain throughout her body, with her hair all loved off, with life seeming like anything other than normal, she finds the familiar. She finds our life in the midst of this nightmare and insists that we live it. It's good that she's the one charting the course. I'm the one that is always ready to assume the fetal position. It has served me well, and I'm not about to veer from a good thing.

Laurie's Journey

So just as I'm going down for the count, Laurie is standing up. Just when I think her body can't take much more, Laurie is suggesting that we get the bikes tuned up and go out for a ride. Just when I think that it might be time to give in for a bit, to encourage her to take a break, I look at her and am reminded that this is Laurie Roth we're dealing with. She doesn't give up, and she sure doesn't give in. I'm reminded of another favorite refrain: "U can't touch this!" Laurie stands; Laurie fights; Laurie wins. Psst . . . hey cancer, keep this in mind: Laurie does not lose! Amen.

Tomorrow we'll walk into the cancer center. I'll be dragging my feet, fumbling with my keys, staring directly into the sun so I have something to blame for the tears in my eyes. Our girl? She'll walk confidently and calmly through the doors and back into a chemo chair. She'll receive all five bags of medicine and thank our nurse as she administers each one. She'll talk to people in the room, making them feel better, feel happier, feel so much more comfortable. Her quiet serenity brings calm to the chaos every single time. I will look around and see people looking at her, being warmed by her grace, drawn to her smile, inspired by her strength. I'll nod knowingly, because that's what she does for me. I know that in Laurie, they are seeing the light at the end of their tunnel, the light that God sent to illuminate the dark days, the light that I am privileged to be alongside every day. That's what I'm talking about: this is livin'!

As always, we'll keep you posted and let you know how the champ does after chemo. Please know that we continue to be so buoyed by your love. Thank you for your continued prayers and all of your positive energy channeled toward a great response in Laurie's body to kick cancer to the curb. You truly are our lifelines, our bright lights, our lifesavers.

Tough Week; Tougher Champ
August 6, 2012

As predicted, the past few days have not been fun ones. They've been nothing that anyone would choose to experience, and yet Laurie knows there is no avoiding them. The side effects are speed bumps in her road to victory. Each ugly one of them has to be endured so that what we have dared hope, dared dream, dared pray for will actually happen: that she will have her scan and it will give her good news. Actually, not good news, GREAT news!

She's had a myriad of side effects, all pretty familiar, yet none getting friendlier the more we get to know them. In fact, the phrase "familiarity breeds contempt" is pretty apropos right now. But Laurie faces the side effects gracefully, not contemptuously. Her tongue swells and makes it painful to talk, her skin hurts, her body aches. Yet she chalks it up as par for the course. She watches her nails turn odd colors, sees red EKG-like lines running through them, and feels the pain that even a simple touch can bring. Yet she's thankful that her nails have not fallen off. She has backaches and chest aches and you-name-it aches. Yet she constantly reminds me that it could be so much worse.

Instead of debating her, I stand in awe of her. I'm in awe that Laurie can continue to be beat up but never beat down. In awe that if I do get her to rest, it's her style of resting: sitting up in the living room, and not for more than thirty minutes. (Clearly, my idea of resting and Laurie's are way different!) In awe that she doesn't cry, doesn't complain, doesn't whine. So I do all those things for her. After all, what are sidekicks for?

But I'm so in awe of her that this weekend I actually asked her how she does it. It was a tough weekend, a trying weekend, one that made me tear up just watching her work through the "cure." When I saw her visibly wince in pain from simply rubbing her own arm, I looked at her and asked, "How do you do it?" She looked at me and, in her constant, selfless way, simply shrugged me off. But I was not letting her off the hook. I needed to have the mystery solved. As valid as my theory is—that she is a superhero with an invisible cape—I needed to hear from her how she actually does it. She looked at me and said, "This is my way of controlling this situation. If I give in to these stupid side effects, then I could get depressed, and then it wins." I broke into a huge smile. It was what I thought all along: Laurie Roth does not lose! Whew!

Laurie and I have story after story of her winning, me losing. While this is not my proudest statement, it is a true one. My personal favorite is from a time shortly after we met, when we decided to play a little tennis. The match started in fairly nice temperatures, but droned on, and soon it was one hundred degrees out. I was up a point, but down a thousand electrolytes. My face was red as a tomato, and I was basically crawling around the court, begging to stop. Laurie? She was trotting around like it was balmy and seventy. I don't think she had even broken a sweat. And she was definitely not leaving until she won—which she did. She won; I lost. She won; I was delirious, hallucinating, and calling for my mommy. She won; I had to be helped to the car—by Laurie. Convinced that I should be taken straight to the hospital for hydration purposes, I was astounded to hear Laurie chirp, "Hey, want to go get some landscaping and plant some flowers?" I'm not making one word of any of this up.

My point is not to humiliate myself (and yet I just did). My point is that this is what Laurie will do to cancer. She will beat it AND rub its nose in it. She doesn't need a cape to be a superhero. She simply is one. And cancer will never, ever see her sweat. In fact, it will never know what hit it, but it will never forget how hard she did.

When God put the finishing touches on Laurie, He must have sat back and said, "Oh, this is a good one. You can't break this one!" God deserves a big ol' high five for his creation of Laurie. As He knew we would need her to do, she shows us all how to face adversity, stare down the monsters, and live. So at this house, that's what we do. Pity parties are on hold, as are whining and complaining. (Darn it, because I am really partial to those last two.) Instead, we are living. Amen to that!

So here we go, working through this week and looking to next week. Next Monday, August 13, is Laurie's PET scan. We then have an appointment to get the results, hot off the presses, on Wednesday, August 15. We are being bold and hopeful and prayerful that significant improvement will be seen in this scan. The chemo is certainly taking the good stuff, so we pray that it is taking the bad stuff too. We will let you know as soon as we know. Please keep Laurie tucked deep in your heart, in your positive places, in your prayers. You give us both amazing strength and comfort just by being with us on this journey. Thank you, beautiful lifesavers!

Scanxiety
August 13, 2012

We arrived at the Community Cancer Center bright and early to prepare for the PET scan. The way this test works is that Laurie has to fast beforehand, drink plenty of water two hours before, and get injected with a radioactive glucose material. We wait for ninety minutes for the glucose to move through her system. Then the scan begins.

From a pain standpoint, this scan is on the easier side for Laurie, if you don't count the ninety minutes she has to sit there listening to me fill dead air. She feigns interest in her iPad, even though the connection is spotty. She looks at a *Better Homes and Gardens* magazine from 2008. She begins to count the ceiling tiles, then finally knows that she might as well give in. It's time to hear about my family's trip to California, and she is just going to have to suffer through it. That spellbinder takes us right up to Ryan (our PET scan tech) arriving at our door, at which point Laurie nearly runs through it. It's not excitement for the scan, it's pure relief that she gets to leave my trip down memory lane.

I know that it's going to take about thirty minutes for Laurie to have the scan, so I settle into the library and begin to pray. She belongs to God first and the rest of us second. God is well aware of the tough months she has faced and how it would be great for her to have earned some good news on Wednesday. But He also knows I'm a nagger, so I tell Him anyway. He is also very aware that she is the strongest person I know, but that even the great Laurie Roth needs a little downtime and ease of mind. I throw it out there anyway. And He has surely heard before what she means to me, what she does for this world, and that there's no better person for Him to shine His light on. But I work it in again for the ten thousandth time.

So here we go. As Laurie and I have talked this weekend, we have reminded ourselves that she's done all she could have done leading up to this day. When the recommendation from Northwestern was one oral chemo with fewer side effects, she upped the ante and took not just the two pills two times a day, but the other mean chemo in an IV every three weeks. When the side effects got so tough that I thought maybe we should take a break, she stood her ground and fought through each and every one. When she could have rested, she kept fighting. Now all we can do is pray, be positive, and be secure that all she has done has been enough.

That's not to say that we don't have moments of scanxiety—a new term for the anticipation of the results. We most certainly do. After all, anxiety and worry are two of my BFFs, but I'm working hard to ignore them. I'm working hard at focusing on Laurie, and every time I do that, I feel nothing but confidence. I've said it dozens of times: there's a fighter in Laurie that fools most people. This gracious, peaceful person who extends kindness and thoughtfulness to all who walk alongside her is one tough scrapper. And that scrapper is my golden ticket to confidence. She will fight her way out of anything. I saw that fighting spirit the first time we went through this, and I watched with complete amazement. I watch it this time with even more awe. Where it comes from, I have no idea. I just know that I never want to be on the other end of it. Fight, Laurie, fight! Just not with me—there's really no sport in fighting with this wimp anyway.

So fight she does, and as I always like to visualize, cancer is crying over in the corner. Cancer has been pummeled and beaten down, and the one-two punches Laurie delivers every time she takes her chemo are making it run like the wind out of her body, out of her life, out of our beautiful world.

Our beautiful world is made up of all of you beautiful souls. Your love and support keep us bolstered, keep us smiling, keep us loved. You are our lifesavers and our army of angels, keeping us strong, keeping us loved, keeping us safe.

Can I Get an Amen?
August 15, 2012

Today was the day we received the PET scan results. Today was the day that we have been thinking about, and we thought of every possible outcome and every possible result. It has been a time of guarded hopefulness, looking on the bright side of what is more often a very dark tunnel, optimistic dreams shrouded in reality of the overall scary situation. My daily prayer was for just a little good news.

My goodness, how God delivers. We didn't get just a little good news, we got a LOT of good news. In fact, we got news that Dr. M. called amazing, incredible, stunning. We got news that he gave to us with a grin a mile wide! We got news that has "miracle" written all over it.

Liver tumors have shrunk in half. Significant reduction in the lung. Right breast tumor reduced. Significant reduction in spot on spine. NO EVIDENCE of disease in neck, mammary, and chest lymph nodes!

Hallelujah! Amen! Thank you, Jesus! Thank you, army of angels who have faithfully prayed and positively thought for our girl! You're not Laurie's Lifesavers for nothing! You're the best of the best!

And can we get a round of applause for our champ? She has done the heavy lifting of three rounds of chemo, terrible side effects, and ongoing pain. She has gotten into the ring, kept punching, and kept fighting, and today we found out that she kept winning! That image of cancer cowering in the corner? It all came true today with these results. Cancer is cowering; cancer is the one crying; cancer is up against the ropes, and Laurie just keeps punching. That's our girl!

Let me tell you how incredible this is. As Dr. M. described, typically at this stage of the game, the best you can hope for is to see some stabilization of the disease—that while it hasn't shrunk, it hasn't grown either. He called it a cancer plateau, and unfortunately, you don't always see that, even with this aggressive treatment. But that's what he was shooting for. To have *significant reduction* is awesome! To have *no evidence of disease* where it had significantly been is absolutely astounding! In fact, I think Laurie took "hammer time" to a whole new dimension! I'm thinking God took the hammer in His own hands and pounded cancer a few times too!

And the hammer is going to have to keep coming down. While it would be nice if Laurie didn't have to have another chemo, it is clearly working, and we can't stop the train now. This is the bittersweet piece for Laurie. Words could never capture her elation over the PET scan results. She is so thankful, so relieved, so very happy. But the chemo must resume, so the fighter stays in the ring.

Our champ has to climb back into the ring for at least two more rounds, maybe three. Her body is weary and already beat up, so we worry what will happen after one more round, let alone three. We asked if we could take a break, just do the oral, ride this happy train of good news from the scan for a while. Dr. M. wasn't budging. He knows a recipe for success when he sees it: Laurie plus chemo equals TKO. In fact, he used a word that we hadn't heard before: remission. If Laurie's body keeps having the results with the next two or three rounds that we have seen after the first three, we're not just talking disease management, we're talking full-blown remission! Now that's what I'm talking about!

So, proving that there truly is no rest for the weary, next Thursday we will sit down and Laurie will have the IV hooked up with our new best friend, Taxotere. She'll begin her run with Xeloda, twice a day for fourteen days. As has been the history, she'll have some really hard days that will take their toll. But we will face them with the knowledge that the chemo is working, that cancer is cowering, that Laurie is winning. We will face the hard days knowing that the light at the end of the tunnel is glowing so brightly, so brilliantly, so beautifully. We will face those days with your love and support, your prayers and your positive energy, your parachute pants and pink hammers! We will face those days, and we will live.

From the bottom of our grateful, thankful hearts, thank you for being in our corner, on our path, on this journey. What blessings you are, you pack of lifesavers, you! AMEN!

But This Was Supposed to Be the Good Week . . .
August 23, 2012

As I've mentioned before, Laurie gets one pretty good week a month during treatment. She gets her treatment, she has ten to fourteen tough days, and then for about five to seven days she feels okay. Her energy level is up, her appetite is back, her smile is somehow even brighter than usual. Unfortunately, she didn't get that good week this last time. Nope. Our champ was knocked for a loop with an ear infection, sore throat, and sinus problems. "But this was supposed to be our good week" was our mantra. It didn't make things easier, but to commiserate felt a little better.

We were riding the high of the awesome PET scan results. Knowing that the treatment was working made us both (made us ALL) feel better. We were going over the actual results word for word when Laurie mentioned that her ear was kind of hurting. We brushed it off—after all, we had PET scan results to celebrate! By the next morning, we had a call in to Katie, our nurse, explaining the symptoms of what appeared to be a full-blown infection in Laurie's ear, nose, and throat. An antibiotic was called in; we got it started—and it barely made a difference. In fact, almost every night Laurie awoke with excruciating pain in her ear, radiating into her neck and throat. We were up for a few hours each night, nursing it along with pain meds, ear drops, a heating pad, and lots of repeating of "But this is our good week."

Another antibiotic was called in, and we started that this past Monday. We thought that although we had lost a few days of our good week, we still had four more days to enjoy before the treatment started again. Even though the treatment loomed in front of us, we thought if we could get even four good days, we would take them. We could do this. Sure we could . . .

Until at 1:30 a.m. Tuesday night, when Laurie awoke in terrible pain again. Keep in mind, she doesn't complain. She has a ridiculously high pain tolerance. She muscles through the worst of anything and never, ever grumbles, whines, or cries. Those are my go-to guys, not Laurie's. And yet, Tuesday at 1:30 a.m., heating pad to her ear, face wrought with pain, she whispered to me, "I'm not sure how much more of this I can do." Bless her heart. Bless her very brave, very strong, but so very tired heart.

I was reminded of the movie *Toy Story*, when Woody looks at all the toys in the face of chaos and says, "Don't panic! This is no time to be hysterical!" And Hamm the piggy bank looks at him with complete terror and says, "This seems like the perfect time to be hysterical!" I'm typically more Woody than Hamm. I don't panic, I don't really do hysterical. Yet hearing Laurie essentially say she may be at her breaking point, seeing her so very worn out, so very beat up, in so much pain, and feeling so frustrated that we had not turned the corner with this new antibiotic, I was Hamm—it really did seem like a good time to be hysterical.

Instead, I looked at Laurie and told her that she had come too far, that we had gotten news too good, that this infection would pass. I prayed to God above and called in all our angels in heaven to heal her, to hold her tight and to let her know that she could do it. We had two more days of our "good" week, and I asked for her to be able to enjoy even just one of them. Just one to reward her for all twenty-one rotten ones before. Just one so that she would walk back into the cancer center, sit down, take the toxin, and look forward to our next good week.

So today, with one good day in her back pocket, she walked into the cancer center, took the toxin, and we're already making plans for our good week. After all, she's the champ, she's my superhero, she's Laurie Roth. She does what doesn't seem possible, she faces the beast (that we now know comes in the form of earaches and infections), and she puts up her pink dukes and fights. Cancer tried hard to knock her down this past round. Yet look who's still standing! It's Laurie standing, and cancer has to be cowering, knowing that it didn't break her. In her invisible Wonder Woman cape, with her brave smile beaming, and showing such amazing grace, Laurie stands. Maybe this is going to be our good week.

Laurie will get her white blood cell booster shot tomorrow, and then we go see Dr. M. in about ten days. Overall, her other blood work looks good, but they are concerned about the state of her fingernails. The Taxotere is doing quite a number on them, although they have yet to fall out. I cringe even as I type the possibility of her nails falling out! A hangnail sends me running for the painkillers, so the thought of her nails actually falling out makes me lie down. Please pray that we move forward through this round without infection, with fingernails in place, and that same brave spirit embodying our champ, who is patiently waiting for her good week.

Thank you to each of you. Your cards continue to pour in. Your calls arrive, as do your emails and your texts. They are covered in love, and therefore, so are we. You're our army, our lifesavers, our lifelines.

Grading on a Curve
September 4, 2012

We had our visit with Dr. M. today, and Laurie's blood work looks "beautiful," to quote our good doctor. And in my opinion, Laurie's blood work is as beautiful as she is. I've always suspected that she's as beautiful inside as she is outside, and this blood work simply confirms it. Her platelets are at a good level, her red blood cells even better, and her white blood cells are actually kind of sticking around this time—how nice of them! Dr. M. was pleased, so we were too.

As weeks go, this was a pretty darn good one, at least in Laurie's manner of measuring—not so much mine. Laurie may be the teacher in the family, but I think I'm a much tougher grader in terms of what is a good day and what is not. And although Laurie has been an amazing sport about her week, I will tell you that it has been a tough one. One that I would have handled with not nearly as much grace and perseverance, and more than likely with a lot of whining and writhing around on the floor. Laurie has

Laurie's Journey

pride and a high tolerance for pain; I have absolutely no shame and—well, I think that says it all.

Let me outline what Laurie has dealt with, and let's see how you would grade it. Her fingernails are not wanting to stick around for the end of the story. Instead, one came completely off (collective cringing can now begin), and that seemed to give all the others permission to come close to doing the same. Who knew that fingernails were such followers? Anyway, they are painful beyond description. I know this because when I see Laurie bump them on a door, a seat belt, or a shoelace, she winces and audibly moans in pain. So while Laurie would give this side effect her proverbial, good-natured "pretty good week" assessment, I say that it's a bad one, and I grade this an F minus.

She has also developed a serious rash on both hands and both forearms. It is itchy, red, and feels like the worst sunburn of your life. Lotion helps a little bit, but mostly everything else just makes it more painful. It hurts just to look at it. Laurie's take on the rash: "It could be worse." Um, no . . . it probably couldn't be worse. So in my grade book, this is also an F minus.

And then all the other familiar characters rolled in this week too—lack of appetite, headaches and body aches, mouth sores and blisters. When I say "lack of appetite," I mean food is not Laurie's friend. Chemo hasn't brought nausea, but it has changed food to the point that it seems worthless to eat it. You have to understand that we are your go-to folks for eating. Historically, we love food; we are the guinea pigs to try a recipe on, and we will eat your food and truly believe that you really are the next Food Network star. But not now. Right now, bland is beautiful—no, not really, not so much. To that I say thank you, Smoothie King—we should buy stock in you for all of our many runs to your blenders! Lest I sound bitter about bland, let's hear Laurie's take on all of this: "At least I didn't get an earache this time." Really? Apparently, that's our new barometer. But I'll be generous and grade on a curve, because I too am thankful that the earache stayed away. I'll give all those side effects a D.

Now, how about Laurie's personal grade in all of this? She herself gets an A plus plus plus—plusses to infinity! As a patient, as an inspiration, as an amazing person faced with the challenge of her life, there aren't enough A plus plusses to put after her name in the grade book. It's her peaceful, graceful, ridiculously strong nature that earns her top honors. In fact, in the world of honorary degrees, Laurie earns a magna cum laude for her smile in the face of danger, her ability to conquer the monster, and her unwavering willingness to show all of us how to survive this thing called life.

So the perfect pupil walks back into the chemo room next Thursday, September 13. We'll sit down, Laurie will take the poison, and we will pray and hope and dare to dream that it will find its way to every bad seed that cancer has tucked in the dark corners of her body. We will look around and truly believe that we have it pretty darn good compared to the others in the room. Not only do we have a wonderful life, but our life is filled to the brim with blessings. It's filled to the brim with you. We find it hard to believe that there is any better support network, a better band of lifesavers, another army of angels so strong, so comforting, so heaven-sent. You bring peace to our world every day, right when we need you to the most. You are so good! You're A plus plus plus too!

Thank you to each of you for all of your love and support each and every day. Our champ is going strong, and it's your prayers and your positive energy that bring her comfort, bring her strength, and always bring her love. From the bottom of our very humble hearts, thank you.

For Good
September 9, 2012

A dear friend recently sent us a song when we were midstream in these dark waters. The song is "For Good" from the musical *Wicked*. The play is kind of the prequel to *The Wizard of Oz* and tells the story of the good witch Glinda and the not-so-good witch Elphaba. "For Good" is a duet by the two witches conveying that great relationships change our lives. Our friend said that it reminds her of Laurie and how inspired she is by Laurie's strength. I couldn't agree more! I've always known that my life was and is changed for the better since the minute Laurie allowed me to be her sidekick. I also know that because I am so very privileged to even know Laurie, my world has been changed for good.

Yesterday was another one of those days when our lives were not just changed for the better, but changed for good. It was Race for the Cure day here in Bloomington. Our loyal team of Laurie's Lifesavers followed a ragtag yellow noodle (no, not me—a yellow pool noodle artfully twisted with wire into the shape of a ribbon, with "Laurie's Lifesavers" lovingly scrawled on it by none other than Tina K.). A few of our lifesavers ran the 5K race; most walked the one-mile route. Some of our lifesavers veered off and did the 5K walk, which I can only assume was an accident, since we are not prone to acts of overexertion. Some of you were not there in person, but you were certainly there in spirit. All in all, Laurie's Lifesavers clocked some good distance, shared deep hugs and great laughs, and brightened the spirits of this lowly captain and our lovely honoree, Laurie.

As if that wasn't enough, we then headed over to Killarney's Irish Pub in Bloomington for a fundraiser in Laurie's honor, with proceeds going to the Community Cancer Center, where Laurie gets her treatment. I am reminded of the words attributed to Margaret Mead: "Never doubt that a small group of thoughtful, committed citizens can change the world. Indeed, it is the only thing that ever has." From a small group of friends and family in our world, dedicated to "doing something" to help us on this journey, blossomed a spectacular event that is slated to raise thousands of dollars for people who cannot afford cancer care. At last count, the funds donated were close to $8,500, with more on the way. Can I get an AMEN?

To say that we are overwhelmed is an understatement. In fact, I think I could search and search and never quite find the words to convey how amazingly thankful we are for all that was put in place for us yesterday. The funds raised will be godsends for those in need; the spirits raised in our two hearts by the outpouring of love and support for us will remain with us forever. The pub was busy all afternoon with people coming in, people staying, people buoying us with wondrous love and support. All of you who were there yesterday or played a part, who donated food or time or money, who were with us in person and with us in your hearts for this amazing event—each and every single one of you has changed our lives for good.

As the song says, because we've known you, you will stay with us like a handprint on our hearts. Isn't that a beautiful sentiment? And it captures exactly how we truly feel. Through these days and nights of pain and side effects, of apprehension over this test or that scan, of prayers and pleadings from so many mouths to God's dear ears, we have felt your hands on our hearts. Through struggles and into triumphs, through paralyzing fear to jumps for joy, through unsteady worries to unwavering support, your hands have been on our hearts. God's hands, your hands, all the hands of all the angels that we have in heaven have left their handprints on our hearts. You are the hands that comfort, support, and love us. How very blessed we are to have each hand on our two hearts.

So when our champ and her trusty sidekick walk into the chemo room this coming Thursday, we will visualize looking from the front door of Killarney's to its far back wall and seeing a sea of faces filling that pub to the brim. These beautiful faces were all there for us. We will walk in with the memory of a small group of friends and family hatching an idea to make this road easier for us (and ultimately others), spending countless hours getting donations, planning the food, planning the fundraiser and every last perfect aspect of it. We will walk in with our spirits at an all-time high, thanks to wonderful people who are all changing our world not just for the better, but for good.

As you listen to the song, please know that although it is easy to think of Laurie as you hear it, we think of you when we listen. From the bottom of our thankful, overwhelmed, and grateful hearts, thank you.

Five Down, One to Go!
September 13, 2012

Today was the day when Laurie completed her fifth chemo session—let's give our champ a round of applause and a hearty AMEN! Be proud of your girl—she took it like the fighter that she is. Champions don't back down from adversity, even though every fiber in their bodies is telling them to run away and not look back. Champions stare the enemy down and make sure that it blinks first. Champions sit in chemo chairs and take the toxin, because the only option is life. It's easy to see why the word "champion" is synonymous with Laurie.

But as you can well imagine, Laurie wanted to be just about anywhere other than the cancer center today. She had even attempted to schedule that gallbladder surgery she's been meaning to have, as well as a root canal and double knee replacement. She wanted to be ANYWHERE other than where our car was heading. It's hard to walk back into the cancer center when you not only know what is coming, but you know the week that you are leaving behind. We've had an amazing week, completely carried by the awesome Race for the Cure and the hugely successful fundraiser in Laurie's honor. As we got closer to today, we kept reminding each other to "think of last Saturday," "visualize that jam-packed room," and "revel in the love of all our angels." And we did. We truly did.

Until today. It had nothing to do with the outpouring of love that we received last week, over the last four months, and over all the yesterdays of this journey. Instead, it was truly about today. Today meant that the side effects we had gained some distance from would be back with a vengeance. Today meant that no matter what Laurie had conquered before, she'd have to battle all over again. Today meant that Laurie would have to put up her very tired dukes, wearily climb back in the ring, and go another long round with cancer. Today seemed almost too hard.

And as God always does, he put angels in our path, right when we needed our angels the most. All of you reading this, all of you sharing this, all of you praying about this are our angels. Some of you came in emails, some came in cards, some came in texts. Some of today's angels came in the form of friends and their pets.

Laurie's Journey

It is no secret that Laurie lives her life to be in the company of dogs. This is no reflection on the love she feels for all of us, but she loves dogs and they love her. Whether it is a dog that is lucky enough to live with Laurie or a dog that she has met even for a minute, a bond quickly forms, and love is born! Today was no exception.

Today, with the triple threat of Taxotere, Xeloda, and Zometa looming in front of her, Laurie took a big heaping dose of canine comfort. She of course has our two dogs, Journey and Harbour. These two would be very content to spend every minute of every day simply sitting in front of Laurie, staring at her with complete adoration. In their eyes, I am mincemeat compared to Laurie. To anyone who knows me, it will come as no surprise that I am hardly the alpha of the pack. Quite the contrary. I am the fun mom, the one who plays and never disciplines, the one they never have to mind and with whom there is not one single rule that cannot be broken. In short, I am so low in the pecking order that I think they think I'm the runt of the litter. But it is Laurie who hangs the moon for them. And I completely understand why.

After spending most of the morning enjoying a Journey and Harbour lovefest, Laurie ran over to the home of our friends Lisa and Lisa to see their three dogs. All of them are adorable, and one of them is a fourteen-week-old yellow Labrador puppy named Gus. Gus comes fully packed with floppy ears, innate cuteness, and puppy breath—a perfect recipe for lightening a mood. He and his doggy siblings gave Laurie good love and many laughs. They kept her spirits bright for most of the morning.

Laurie left Gus and company and came home just as I was getting home from work to take her to the cancer center. Her face broke my heart. Without saying a single word, her face begged me to take her anywhere but to chemo. Her face, and the tears coming down her beautiful cheeks, told me that the champ was on the ropes—not giving in, but not so sure about going another round today. Knowing my role as trusty sidekick, I knew what I had to do. I had to be inspiring; I had to be motivating; I had to be positive. This, unfortunately, would require speaking, and try as I might, I could not voice one audible word. Instead, all I could do was turn to Laurie and match her tear for tear. At that moment, looking at that beautiful face, with her hair loved off, her nails falling out, and her body so tired, I cried. I quickly realized that I really needed to buck up. So I pulled myself together and reminded both of us that Laurie Roth doesn't lose and we need to keep the beast on the run. Nasty chemo number five had to go in and complete its search-and-destroy mission so we could get on with our wonderful, amazing life. She reluctantly agreed, and off to chemo we went.

We pulled into the lot, Laurie not even wanting to open her eyes as we parked. I suggested that she was definitely going to want to see who was there to greet her. She looked up to see our sweetheart of a friend, Jill, in the parking lot of the cancer center with her two dogs, Clover and Roy. The part of the story that you have to be told is that Roy O'Flaherty and Laurie Roth have had a long love affair. And today, Roy needed to see his girlfriend, and his girlfriend needed to see him. So his very thoughtful mom drove Roy and his sister over to the parking lot right before we arrived, to serve as Laurie's welcoming committee, cheerleaders, and pep band! The many tears that had filled my eyes on the drive over turned to tears of pure joy. I saw Laurie's face go from worry and dread to a full-blown Laurie Roth light-the-world-up smile. It was a perfectly timed, perfect present—for both of us.

With doggie kisses and wagging tails cheering us on, we walked into the cancer center. The very door Laurie didn't think she could go through, the one I didn't know how I'd get her to go in, didn't seem so hard to open now. Laurie's step was lighter, her smile brighter, and we even laughed a few times in the waiting room. We couldn't stop being thankful for the angels on our path, four-legged and two-legged alike. They called her name, and up we stood. Hello, hammer time!

So now the triple threat is going through our champ. The next seventy-two hours will not be fun, and Sunday will more than likely be the worst. I'm an optimist by nature, but the last four bouts with chemo have taught me that history will repeat itself. Laurie will feel all the old side effects and probably even a few new ones. It's chemo, not Children's Tylenol, looking for every single cancer cell. The problem is that it takes the good ones too. She'll feel puny, she'll be vulnerable to germs, and she won't have one ounce of appetite. But in true Laurie Roth fashion, she won't lie down, she won't give in, and I assure you, she won't give up. This is a fight for which she stays on her feet, jabbing and punching, mowing and vacuuming, laughing and smiling. I ask her the same question every day: "Did you ever know that you're my hero?" I resist the urge to belt out Bette Midler's beautiful song—after all, Laurie has suffered enough, so she sure shouldn't have to hear me sing another show tune (the operative word being "another"). But it is her graceful, quiet strength that inspires me, that motivates me, that melts me. Those who have seen her smile in the face of this wolf at our back door know exactly what I'm talking about.

Please keep her in your prayers. Chemo is cumulative, so nasty number five is going to give us a run for our money. Our nurse today informed Laurie that her nails look "about as painful and as awful as any nails" she has seen in her many years in oncology. While I've mentioned that Laurie has a competitive side, I don't think this was a contest that she meant to win. The nerves in her face are burning and causing unfathomable pain in her mouth. And yet she smiles. She smiles, and when she does, my world, our world, brightens and hope springs eternal. As long as we have you and we have hope and we have Laurie's smile, we are unbeatable!

Thank you for all of your love and support. Thank you for being right where we need you, right when we need you the most. Thank you for sharing your lives, your love, and our story so that all the prayers and positive thoughts of God's people carry Laurie forward through nasty number five. We have set our sights on remission and won't stop until we get it. We're in it to win it, folks! Please make that your prayer.

She Was Built to Not Break
September 21, 2012

So here we are, eight days past nasty number five, and boy, has it been a doozy! Laurie has had all the old familiar side effects—body aches, skin aches (yes, skin aches), horrible nail issues, and even worse mouth sores. While we had seen mouth sores before, we hadn't seen them to this degree. In fact, when Laurie showed me her mouth sores and her tongue riddled with blisters, all I could do was shudder and lie down. That's not nearly as helpful as I had hoped, so I'm going to have to think of a new response.

Along with all the old familiars came either a cold or some allergies. It started with a slightly scratchy throat that turned into a really sore throat and then something that settled completely in her head—nose stuffed, eyes watering, you know the drill. Poor thing—so weak from nasty number five, and now her body had to spend energy coughing, wheezing, and sneezing. I bet you're probably thinking that at least this cold or allergy thing might make her lie down and rest. That is so cute that you would think that. It's Laurie, people—she does not lie down!

As we've gone along this week, she has somehow managed to move my hero needle from complete adoration to all-out worship. I've spoken of her grace; I've written of her courage; I've babbled on and on about the great Laurie Roth to anyone who would even act like they were listening. But this week, as she faces down chemo number five, feeling like a wet noodle and still living life as beautifully as she did before that awful dark blob appeared on the pathology screen, I absolutely stand in awe of her.

I picture God making her fifty-one years ago and how He must have smiled, knowing what He was handing down to earth. He put in just the right mix of humor and grace and kindness to make a personality that, once known, would never be forgotten and would always be loved. He blew in a gentle spirit with inner strength and peace that would create a safe haven for all who met her. He knew this world would be hard sometimes, disappointing and challenging, so He gave her empathy, understanding, and the ability to see the best in people and in situations. He knew that someday her hair would be all loved off, so He took His hands and lovingly rounded her little noggin into a perfect egg. He knew that she would pursue a life of teaching children and share her life with a sidekick who acted like a child, so He doubled up on patience and calmness and encouragement.

He molded her into the person who shows up for life even when it would be so easy to mail it in. He gave her feet that can bob and weave and even break into a few smooth dance moves. He gave her hands that gently soothe a soul and fists that fiercely beat cancer into the corner. He made sure that in Laurie we would all see how to live, both in the storms and in the sunshine. There's no doubt in my mind that she simply was built to not break.

And this week proves it. We've faced mouth sores and blisters, skin aches and joint aches, and needling thoughts that maybe nasty number five was going to be the one that made her crumble. Not one day in this entire week has she felt anything close to 100 percent. In fact, we'd be happy with 50 percent. But this is Laurie Roth. Give her even less than 50 percent and she'll take it and run with it—literally. Nasty number five pulled some good punches, wobbled our little Weeble, but look who's standing now? In fact, she's not just standing, she's tapping her toe waiting for me to finish so we can walk the dogs! That's what I'm talking about!

And let's not forget about you, our beautiful lifesavers and angels. You call, you write, you make us laugh, you bolster our spirits with your prayers and positive energy. Thank you. You're cheering on a champion, and we are so close to the finish line! On October 5 we will go for our next chemo, which we are calling our last chemo. That's the goal, that's what we'll settle for, that's what we're shooting for. Please pray for great healing and continued strength in our girl, and pray that hammer time has done the trick!

Homestretch
September 30, 2012

So here we are, entering the homestretch. We've made the turn and we're heading down the straightaway to the finish line. As in most races, the one out in front is tired, especially since she has led the whole way. There have been days when it must have felt like cancer was nipping at her heels, so close she could hear it right behind her. Sometimes it had to seem to Laurie like they were almost neck and neck. That's not how I saw it, though. In my mental image, Laurie is always in the lead, out in front, leaving cancer in the dust. I am a master at creating my own reality, so that is the one I've made and the one that I'm sticking with. I like that image, don't you?

But I know from looking at our girl and watching the race unfold that it's an exhausting race—physically, mentally, and emotionally. It is draining energy from all corners of Laurie's life, and where she digs from to hit the homestretch, I have no idea. All I know is that Laurie runs like there's no tomorrow. My guess, and my very thankful prayer, is that she runs like this so that she can have, and we can have, so many more tomorrows. She runs like the wind, not just for her tomorrows, but for my tomorrows and your tomorrows, for all of us so very lucky to share our lives, our hearts, our world with Laurie Roth. Amen.

Almost to the day, this all began four months ago when we heard the words "Laurie's cancer is back." Those four powerful, life-changing words made our world simultaneously come to a screeching halt and spin wildly out of control. We were thrown into a flurry of tests and scans, biopsies and blood draws, second opinions and sometimes second thoughts. All the while we were trying to get our feet back under us so the beast didn't get one step ahead, not even for a second. The beast can't be in the lead; the beast must always be in the dust.

We then heard scarier words, like "It's in your liver, in the lining of your lung, in a spot on your spine." It seemed like our world became eerily silent and chaotically, deafeningly loud all at the same time. As I was buckling at the knees, Laurie was lacing up her boxing gloves and racing shoes. She chose to take not one, but two really strong, really mean, really harsh chemo drugs. These are the drugs that act more like the enemy than teammates as they attack the good along with the bad. Because of her "helpers," Laurie has felt pain like she has never known, has been beaten up and sucker punched. She has lost her fingernails, her hair has all been loved off, and her body aches from head to toe. It's not called "hammer time" for nothing, folks.

This woman of amazing grace, the softest heart, and the sweetest spirit has not been in the fight to win by a nose. No way. From the minute our world turned upside down, Laurie has been in it to dominate throughout and beat cancer to a pulp. It is pure peace and gentleness that runs through her veins—until she's in a competition. From Scrabble to tennis, from Old Maid to one-on-one basketball, from chemo to cancer, she's in it to win it. I know this from personal experience; apparently cancer had to learn this twice. Our champ is not looking for just a homer; she's knocking it out of the park. She's not looking to win by a nose; she will run it into the ground. She's not waiting for the bell to ring and signal that the fight is over; she's looking to pummel and pound cancer until it waves its teeny-weeny white flag and cries "uncle!" Game over, grand slam, total TKO!

Although I am prone to avoid breaking a sweat, I am told that even champions get weary. As the trusty sidekick of the number one champion of my world, I see my champ getting sick, getting tired, getting sick and tired of all of this. It would be so easy to throw in the towel, to walk away, to try to rebuild our old normal and forget about this new normal that we never, ever chose. And just when I think Laurie is on the brink of waving her own white flag, she stands up, pulls out the vacuum, and gets back into the race, into the fight, and into the lead.

I thank her every single day for putting the poison in to get the cancer out. I thank her every single day for letting our world have the best shot to have the best tomorrows. And I thank God every single day for creating Laurie Roth with the heart of a champion, the spirit of a winner, and the soul of a survivor. She has taken one for the team, and I do not know how I will ever repay her. I just know that as I did in all our yesterdays, I will celebrate her in all of our tomorrows.

Simply Overwhelmed!
October 5, 2012

Since we began this journey four months ago, we have used certain words over and over. Some are suitable for print, and others, well, not so much. In fact, when I think of some words we've spoken, I immediately hear my mom, complete with Canadian accent, remind me that "we don't talk like that, dear." So I'll repeat the ones that my dear mom would approve of—words like "wonderful" and "amazing" and "blessed."

We used those words when we thought of you, dear angels. We used those words when we read your cards, your emails, your texts. We used them in our prayers of thanksgiving for putting us on this journey with the best cheering squad ever assembled. The other word that we used even more often was "overwhelmed." Because more often than not, you overwhelmed us with your love, your support, and your constant care of, and for, both of us.

This week was no exception. Today we used the word "overwhelmed" over and over. Today took "overwhelmed" to an all new level. The texts poured in, the cards flooded the mailbox, a bouquet of gorgeous flowers arrived twenty minutes before we were to leave for the cancer center. What do I always tell you? You arrive right when we need you the most. And arrive you did—in spirit and in person!

Leaving the house today was no easy feat. I was anxious to do so, because I knew who was waiting for us. But Laurie walked around the house as if her feet had been dipped in cement. She was walking so slowly, I briefly thought that she was actually walking backwards. But knowing what she was facing, what was waiting, what she had to do to give us our tomorrows, I could understand why she was walking slower than molasses in January. It was dreary, it was rainy, it was almost as if even Heaven cried that she had to go through this.

But go we did. Before we left, we did all the things that we always do before we leave for chemo day. We did the family prayer with the pets, we packed the chemo bag, and we left the house. We drove two blocks and pulled into the parking lot of the cancer center. As we drove up, we saw a group of more than twenty people standing by the front door, smiling broadly, holding pink balloons. Laurie said to me as we pulled in, "Why are all those people there?" In a panic to keep from spoiling the surprise, I said, "It's probably someone's birthday." Clearly, I'm not a good liar, because in all the days we have been there, I've not once seen a birthday celebrated there. It's the cancer center, not Chuck E. Cheese's.

In an effort to get Laurie to stop asking questions, I floored the car toward the crowd (sorry, lifesavers, but I did). Soon the faces of some of our closest, best friends came into focus—all cheering, all smiling, all holding pink balloons in honor of our champ! In the crowd was Laurie's other boyfriend, Gus—our friends' four-month-old Labrador Retriever that Laurie plans to dognap someday. Nothing like a little dog love to put the icing on the cake! This group of lifesavers cheered for us, hugged us tight, and sent us in to take number six and get the finish line even closer. On this dreary, rainy day, we walked into the cancer center buoyed by the love of wonderful, beautiful people—our people leaving their loving handprints on our hearts.

The fun didn't stop there. We walked up to our pal Tara, the receptionist, who was smiling even more broadly than usual. She declared our lifesavers "amazing" and then handed Laurie a bag of Chips Ahoy cookies with a card from a dear friend named Beth. Beth's card declared Laurie to be one tough cookie, and that gave us even more strength to walk through the doors of the chemo room. So walk we did, walking on air all the way back to the chemo chairs. We sat down, babbling deliriously about how amazing our lifesavers are, not only those outside the center but those with us in spirit, and how very overwhelmed we were with the outpouring of love being showered upon us on a day that had loomed like a hurricane in front of us.

The chemo went in, and Laurie smiled her beautiful smile all around the chemo room, drawing one person after another, myself included, to her energy, her spirit, her strength. We chatted with a dear friend who spent time with us, and we paid it forward with a newbie and her husband sitting down for the first time to fight the fight. And every time we had a break in the action, we said to each other, "Do you believe how wonderful that was?" Completely overwhelmed. But I also knew that being "overwhelmed" was not quite over. I knew that some of Laurie's teacher friends were coming to the cancer center to cheer us OUT the doors, much like we had been cheered IN the doors!

Today of all days, the chemo dripped in at a snail's pace, and we were running horribly behind schedule. At the approximate time that we should have been leaving, I texted the organizer and asked if they were there. Sure enough, these punctual, perfectly timed, wonderful teachers and principals were all assembled outside the doors. I got up to go see them when I was approached by the director of the cancer center, Barb. She knows us and has taken incredible care of us. She also knows that we are loved beyond measure. She walked up to me with a smile as big as the sun and said, "We have the best problem two people could have." She pointed to the front doors of the cancer center, and outside those doors I saw beautiful faces beginning to assemble in perfect cheering formation. I looked back at Laurie getting her chemo, I looked out at the group of lifesavers, and I began to cry. They were tears of pure joy, pure love, pure appreciation. Barb said to me, "Linda, we have to get these poor people out of the rain and into our girl!" We quickly tried to figure out exactly how to do this, but the chemo area was jammed, and bringing over thirty people and one adorable dog named Wrigley in seemed impossible. Then I remembered who we were dealing with: it's Laurie Roth—she can do anything, and her chemo is on wheels!

So with the permission of the head nurse, and with the director of the cancer center pushing Laurie's chemo machine, we walked out to the cheers and applause of many wonderful, beautiful lifesavers from the school district where Laurie taught! We saw faces of some of the dearest friends people are privileged to know. We saw faces smiling and crying and beaming, all for our champ! We saw hands holding pink balloons and ready to hug us tight. We felt the love and support that only a group of comrades can give to one of their own and her sidekick—the sidekick who marvels and humbly appreciates that everyone else is in on the not-so-big secret that this Laurie Roth girl is a being to behold!

To say that we are overwhelmed is an understatement. But when I looked up the definition (because I am that big of a dork), I realized why that word is even more perfect than many of the ones that my mom would never have allowed me to print. The very first definition of "overwhelm" is "to cover completely." Are you smiling too? I bet you are. I bet you know exactly where I'm going with this. I bet you know because you are the reason someone, somewhere, created the word "overwhelm."

Whether you were at the cancer center shivering and standing with pink balloons in your hand or you were there in spirit with pink balloons in your heart, you cover us completely. Whether you call us every day or simply think of us every once in a while and pray "Please, God, take them through this," you cover us completely. Whether you send a card or send your love in spirit, you cover us completely. You cover us completely with pure support, pure comfort, pure love. After all, you're Laurie's Lifesavers, and every single act of love and comfort covers us completely. From the bottom of our very overwhelmed hearts, we thank you.

So here we go. Number six is on its way—on a mission to search and destroy the beast. Number six is on the move, looking in every nook and cranny for even the slightest cell that resembles the monster. Number six is on its way so that soon, our life will look remarkably similar to how it looked four months and one day ago. I'm thinking I have a new lucky number, and that number is six!

To all of you who have said one prayer, thought one positive thought, or fallen on your knees and cried with me, "Not her, not again, please, not Laurie," we love and adore you. You are lifesavers of the highest quality. Every single day, we are thankful that you are in our lives.

The next PET scan will be in about two or three weeks. But we'll be in touch before then. Please know that the love and support you share with us every day, and that you showered upon us today, on this hardest of days, make the next days all the better. Like Laurie has done for me since she first allowed me to be her Tonto, you make both of us better people. I don't think that Laurie Roth can become much better than she already is. But I can assure you, between my Kemosabe and you beautiful lifesavers, I will eventually be the best Tonto ever! And you, you gorgeous, wonderful lifesavers, here with us today and here with us in spirit, completely overwhelm us, completely love us, completely cover us. For that, we will be forever grateful, forever thankful, forever loved.

Laurie's Laughing
October 14, 2012

So here we are, nine days postchemo, and as suspected, all the old familiar side effects are showing up, some so much worse this round than any other. I guess they know that this is their last time in Laurie's body and are determined to go out with a bang. They've never been quiet tenants, so a loud and disruptive goodbye party is par for the course! Maybe even the side effects are celebrating that Laurie survived both the disease and the cure.

We knew when we started on this road that it wasn't going to be a run in the park but would truly be a marathon. Like most races, it wouldn't end soon enough, it would test us, and to win it, we'd have to go the distance. The distance is filled with twists, turns, and uphill battles—tests and scans, scary waits and scarier results, and two chemo drugs called Xeloda and Taxotere that collide in Laurie's body like freight trains crashing head-on.

It is a regimen that requires amazing mental fortitude, great physical strength, and emotional stamina—none of which are my strong suit.

Laurie's Journey

Fortunately for all of us, that's where Laurie shines. She epitomizes putting mind over matter, pulling from her gut, and staying calm in the chaos. She refuses to be a victim, settling for nothing less than being the victor. Despite being in the longest of hauls, taking the strongest of chemo drugs, experiencing almost every single side effect that they warned us about and experiencing them to the nth degree, she's still running. Not *from* cancer—oh, no way. This is Laurie Roth—she runs head-on *into* anything that threatens to be in her way. She is running straight into cancer, bowling it over and leaving it looking for the license plate of the bus that just took it down. She is determined that nothing is going to divide her from this life that she loves; this life that she shares with a silly sidekick, wonderful family, and beautiful friends; this life that she fights every single day to have and to hold from this day forward. Amen. Whew. And a big thank you, Jesus, for building her not to break.

Speaking of family, we added a kitten to ours. Of course we did. Right now, right here, with all that's going on, it seemed like the right time to add a new little being to our world . . . um, not so much. Apparently that's what you do when your plate is overflowing and you have to muster up energy just to put your socks on (I'm talking about me right now, not Laurie)—you decide to bring a little kitten into your family. If you're like I was when Laurie first broached the subject, you're thinking, "Are you kidding me right now?" If you're like me, you are shaking your head, thinking, "Now is really not the right time for a new houseplant, let alone a kitten!" And if you're like me, you give in to Laurie, because she's the boss and she's going to win and she's yet to have a bad idea about adding anything to our life that hasn't made it better. Including this time.

Enter Hobo Jones, an all-black, gold-eyed, four-month-old beautiful kitten. We named him Hobo because he was found out by a farm in the country, and we picture him with a little satchel on his back, patches on his pants, and possibly even a beat-up old hat. See how good Laurie is—give me a mental picture like that, and how can I say no? And in spite of all the reasons I thought we shouldn't adopt a kitten, I'm listening to the exact reason that I'm glad we did: right now I hear Laurie cracking up at one of his antics. Our house is filled with laughter again, and Laurie is leading the refrain.

With blisters on and around her tongue and mouth sores everywhere else, Laurie laughs. With a rash going from her hands up her arms, she plays with Hobo and laughs so hard it makes me laugh. With the chemo draining her of energy, she gets on the floor and becomes Hobo's jungle gym, laughing the whole time. She laughs because Hobo really is funny, filled with such joy and so cuddly that when you're not laughing with him, you're soaking up some of the best love God ever created. Journey and Harbour are in heaven too, enjoying our new addition. They love him and he loves them—something they're really not used to from our other cat, Miss Ali. Speaking of Alicat, the fact that she has not killed or maimed Hobo is a victory. Actually, she's been so good with him that we think she actually, much to her surprise, likes the little guy.

Hobo has brought good life into this house—for every single one of us, but especially for the one who is cracking up at him right now. I mean the one with her hair all loved off, her fingernails hanging by threads, and her body so very beat up everywhere else. Laurie is laughing. Laurie has earned every ounce of this feeling, and to hear her laugh is music to my ears. For all of you who know Laurie's sweet laugh, it's music to yours too. May every day have time devoted to that wonderful, beautiful sound.

We have some specific requests for you, our beautiful lifesavers: prayers and positive energy! They are what you do best, and we are the lucky recipients of your wonderful love every single day. We hope and pray that Laurie's side effects wane, rather than pick up speed, over the next week; that her scan on October 25 is clean and clear and has "REMISSION!" written all over it when we get the results on October 30; that this marathon, this hammer time, this time in the ring, will have been just exactly what was needed to beat the beast and send it running, never, ever to return. Those are our hopes, our prayers, our dare-to-dreams. I hold fast to one vision: Laurie Roth in her pink boxing gloves, arms over her head, and the finish line far behind her! I usually include the theme from *Rocky*, just to put the finishing touches on my vision. Please let that be your vision too.

Thank you for coming to us in your emails, your cards, and your calls. You are our wonderful comforters, sources of strength, and handprints on our hearts. We love and cherish each one of you.

Checking Off the Checklist
October 21, 2012

So if you didn't already know that you're cheering on the absolute strongest champ around, my recap of this week should completely confirm it. As you will remember, the side effects had really taken it up a notch this time. They arrived early, making a lot of noise; they kept their bad behavior up during all hours of the day and night and were showing no signs of leaving. They really were the guests from H-E-double-hockey-sticks!

The day before Laurie's last chemo, we had made a checklist of all the side effects she has experienced on this journey. We listed everything from mouth sores to muscle aches, fatigue to fingernails, skin peeling to skin rashes. We thought it would be powerful to scratch them off the list as each one was done, knowing that Laurie had survived not just the cancer, but also the cure.

Each day came with us hovering over the list, anxiously anticipating scratching off one or maybe even two side effects. Each day ended with the pen unused and the list intact. The side effects weren't leaving. In fact, they appeared to have moved in to stay and even invited their equally ill-behaved relatives! Instead of scratching the side effects off, we found ourselves actually adding to the list. This was going in the wrong direction quickly and was clearly not the symbolism we were shooting for. The list was meant to be more phoenix rising, not *Titanic* sinking!

Every day my prayer was the same: "Dear Lord, please let Laurie begin to feel even just a little bit better. Just a glimmer of hope and sunshine is all she needs." But the rains kept coming, literally and figuratively. The days were cold and rainy and the nights dark and dreary. As this went on and the side effects picked up speed, I began my daily prayer with "Helloooooo, Lord—it's me again. Any chance for a bit less rain and lot more sunshine for our girl?" Hey—God built Laurie overloaded with grace and sweetness, but He spilled far too much sarcasm into me. He knows it, I know it, and we both deal with it. Thankfully, He's a forgiving God who enjoys all of His children, even me.

Meanwhile, our girl was going through it like the champ we know her to be. Was she happy that her mouth was riddled with sores and blisters? Was she tickled pink that she was so tired that she, the great Laurie Roth, actually had to take a thirty-minute nap in the middle of the day? Was she over the moon at the fact that her fingernails and toenails were heading south? No, but not one of those hurdles was going to take her down. They were there for her to get over, get past, and get on with it. She brought the same fighter's spirit to the sixth round that she did to the first. This was her own private hammer time, and she needed to pound cancer into the dust.

It was then that God really should have said to me, "Helloooooo, Linda, it's me again. When will you learn that our girl finds the sunshine in the rain, the joy through the sadness, the light in the darkness? You have forgotten that I built her strong and graceful, courageous and kind, beautiful and brave. I built Laurie Roth to endure, to survive, to live. I built her not to break." Fortunately, God isn't big into the "I told you so." But his message to me was clear.

It became crystal clear two weeks into round six, when we began scratching off the side effects on our list. Mouth sores gone—check! Skin rash gone—check! Fatigue almost gone—close enough—check! Fingernails and toenails—well, they'll come back, and they're not any worse, so—check! The leaf blower is blowing, the vacuum is vacuuming, the house is completely decked out with all of the fall decorations! The chain saw sawing cannot be far behind! Amen!

And yesterday we celebrated birthdays in our house—Laurie's and mine. We were both born on the same date, one year apart. To nobody's surprise, I'm older. My looks give it away, but my actions and behaviors shave off decades. I can't imagine a sweeter time to celebrate life than right now—counting not just the number of years, but the number of breaths, both breaths taken and breaths taken away. Counting not the challenges, but the blessings. Counting not the heartaches, but the handprints. Not surprisingly, we're still counting. Thanks to each of you, each of our blessings, each handprint on our hearts, we will be counting for a long time to come.

The scan is this Thursday, and we get the results on Tuesday, October 30. Let's bombard heaven with prayer and the galaxies with positive energy, all aimed at getting good news! We will let you know as soon as we know. You're our army, our ringleaders, our lifesavers. Thank you for everything!

We got this!
October 29, 2012

One of the hardest things I had to do today was leave home this morning. It's always hard, mainly because I love it here. I love this world that we have created within this little family of ours—this little family that consists of one superhero, her sidekick, two golden retrievers named Journey and Harbour, an ornery but beautiful cat named Ali, and a darling, adorable kitten, new to the fold, named Hobo. From my eyes, it is heaven on earth. God smiled on me when He created this life for me. Every day I leave here reluctantly, but so very thankful. I have been given a family so good that from the second I leave, all I'm wanting to do is get back home. I've said it a thousand times: it is good to be Linda Jones.

Today was certainly no exception. More than usual, I was wanting to stay home. In fact, if you had seen me, you would have wondered who dipped my shoes in cement, why my feet were dragging on the ground, why I was stalling all over the house to avoid walking out the door. Why? Because it simply didn't seem right not to stay home and try to keep Laurie busy as we step back into the not-so-wonderful world of scanxiety. It's a reality show that nobody should ever have to be a part of, and certainly one that should never be viewed alone. Yet here we are, on the eve of receiving the PET scan results—the ones that will tell us whether the last two and a half months of Laurie's fight have really done the trick and sent cancer running for the hills.

Every fiber of every bone in my body wanted to be right where I was—at home, hanging out, following Laurie around and keeping all of us busy. Busy enough to keep us from looking at the clock every five minutes. Busy enough to keep us from feeling like time was actually going backward instead of forward toward tomorrow and our appointment time of 10:30. I thought I might even throw in an impromptu pity party of sorts, when Laurie wasn't looking, just to burn up some time. It had been awhile since I had assumed the fetal position, but I would bet good money that it would come right back to me. It always does.

Just when I thought I should practice my fetal position, I felt a not-so-gentle nudge—a nudge that I can only assume came from my angel mother reminding me of two things: One, she didn't raise a wimp, so get up. And two, God had put together a very strong supporting cast ready to spring into action, so let go and let God. I looked around and saw this beautiful family made up of a superhero and a sidekick, big dogs and little cats, friends and family too many to count, all of whom were going to give us all that we needed to ride this train into tomorrow. As usual, my dear, sweet angel mom was absolutely right.

Journey and Harbour are pure golden retriever love through and through. They know exactly what Laurie needs, right when she needs it—whether it be a paw to hold, a belly to rub, or just soulful brown eyes to sit and have a stare-down with, eyes that look deep into their mom's soul and remind her that she will be just fine. They have been the best medicine, the best nursemaids, the best Florence Nightingales. They have managed to make Laurie's worst days better and her good days amazing.

While we remain convinced that Alicat is half Bengal tiger, she has shown us in the past four months that she is actually all heart. Ali seems to know that when her mom's energy is low, petting and rubbing a beautiful, silky cat might be just what the doctor ordered. We are not fooled into thinking that Ali is enjoying any of it. After all, she has her own bedroom and personal wait staff, so a simple lap is slumming in Ali's world. But she senses that Laurie needs to pet her, needs to sometimes hold her, wants to always have her near. So even Ali gives in and gives her mom a lift through the day, a pleasant surprise, a purrfect way to while away the time.

And Hobo Jones? Well, it turns out that this little barn cat is part court jester and part rodeo clown. He is here purely for distraction, and the timing of his variety show couldn't have been more perfect! He is a mama's boy, and the mama he loves is the one he uses as a jungle gym—Laurie. He cannot get enough of her. If he's not clowning around and getting her to play with him and his vast array of toys, he is asleep in her arms. He knows two speeds: 180 miles per hour and "stop," both of which are thoroughly enjoyed by Mama.

When I turned to leave this morning, I realized that I was leaving our girl in very capable paws. In fact, I could have sworn I heard one of them say to me, "Go on, Mom, we got this." They may have even thrown in a "Don't let the door hit you on the way out," but I might be mistaken. Either way, they did have this. And if they slept, God was awake, and He had this. And don't think I've forgotten about you. We know so well that you had this. You have had us in your thoughts and in your hearts. You have had us on your prayer lists and to-do

Laurie's Journey

lists. You send us cards and texts and emails. You have us, you have this, and we are the very lucky beneficiaries of your good love.

So collectively, it's true: we got this. And now, fourteen hours after thinking I should delay my walk out the door, I say scanxiety, schmanxiety! While we are certainly shooting for nothing but good news, we know the foe is a wily one. From day one, my money has been on Laurie—the unstoppable, unbreakable, undefeatable Laurie Roth. May her heavy lifting these past four months be rewarded tomorrow. She has fought hard, she has fought long, she has fought to win. I pray to heaven above that the victory dance starts tomorrow.

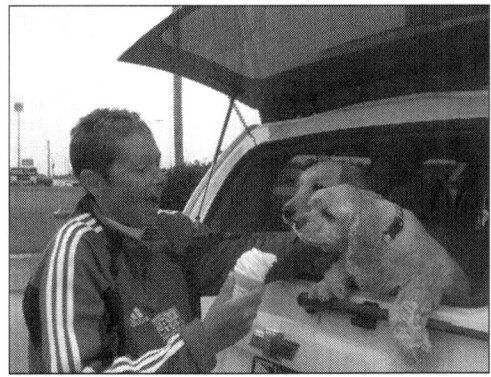

Laurie always found time to spoil the dogs with ice cream.

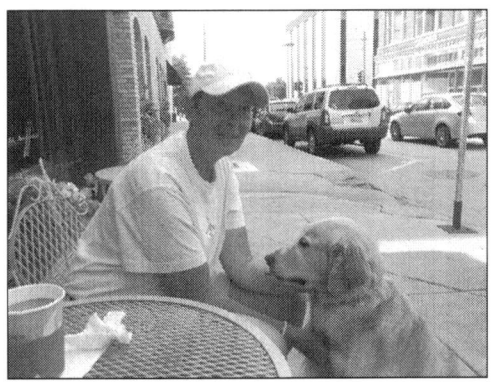

Laurie and Journey at the Farmer's Market.

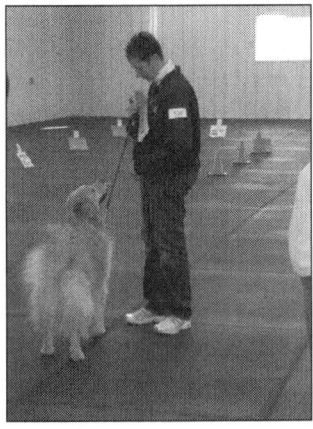

Laurie and Journey earn obedience ribbons.

Laurie's Journey

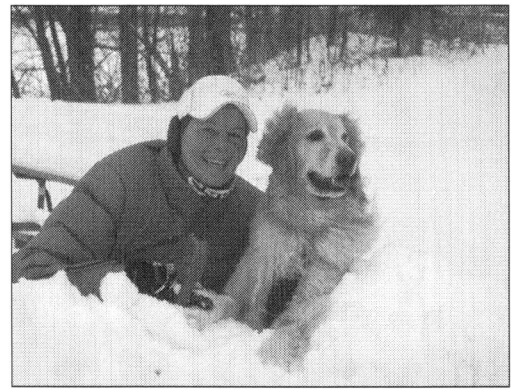

Laurie and Journey playing in the snow.

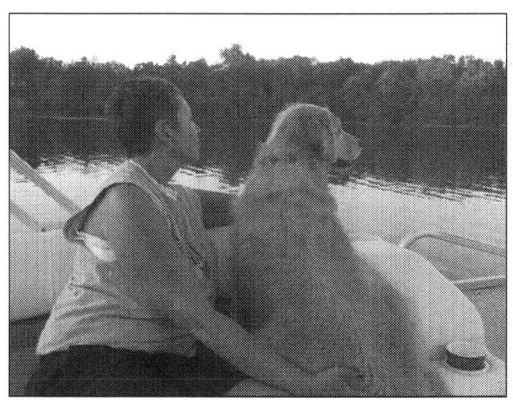

Enjoying a peaceful moment at the lake.

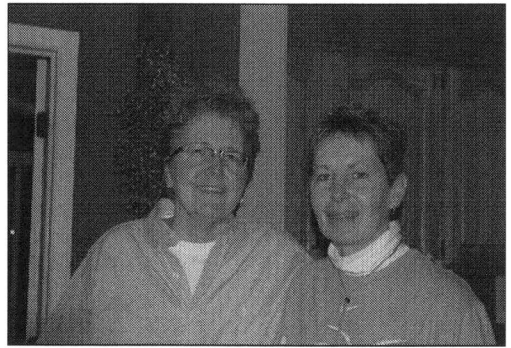

Linda and Laurie winter 2012 after one of the women's basketball games honoring cancer survivors.

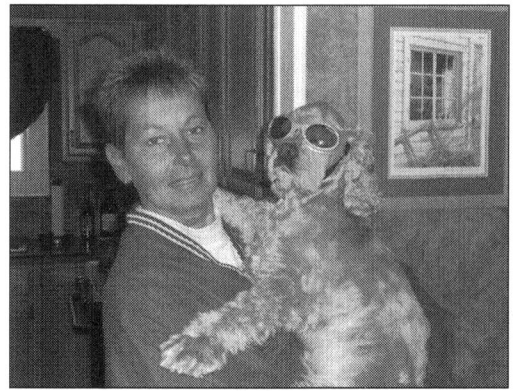

Laurie and Max hamming it up for the camera.

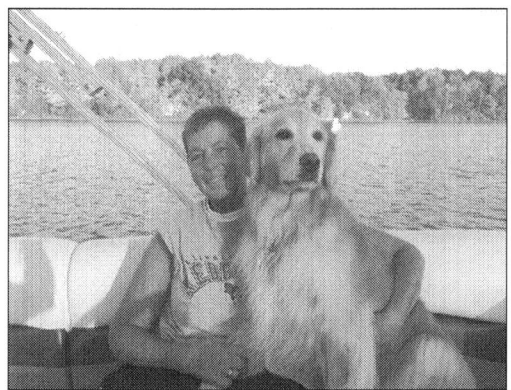

Laurie and Journey enjoying total bliss on the boat.

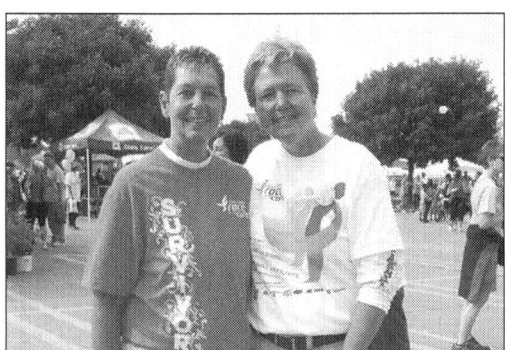

Laurie and Linda after the Race for the Cure.

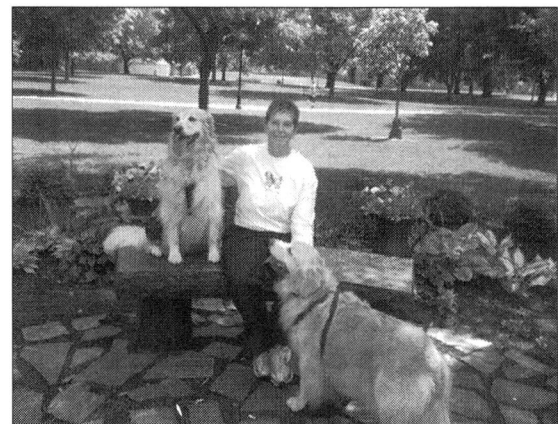

Laurie, Journey and Harbour on the local college campus.

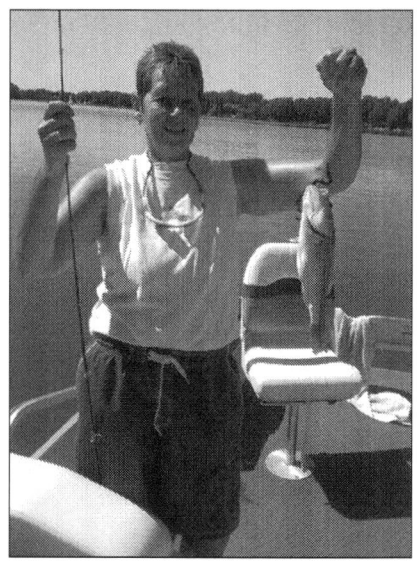

This was a great day fishing capped off by a big catch!

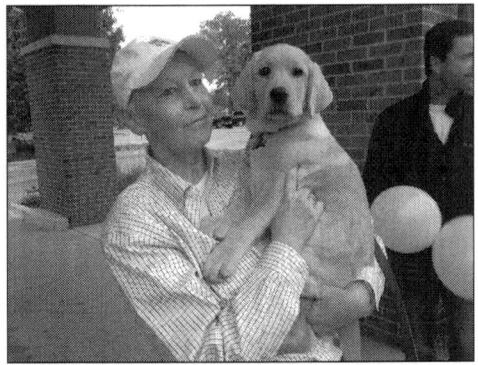

Laurie and her puppy pal Gus - Fall 2012.

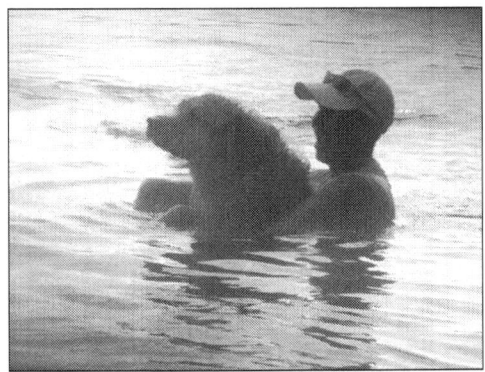

Laurie and Harbour go for a swim.

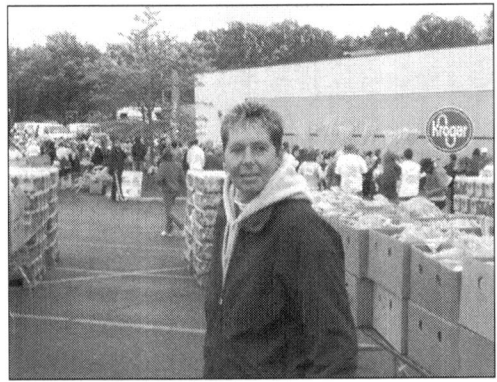

Laurie checking out all the prep for the Race for the Cure.

Laurie's Journey

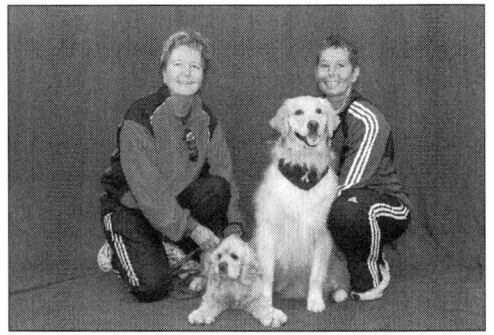

A family photo of Linda, Max, Journey and Laurie.

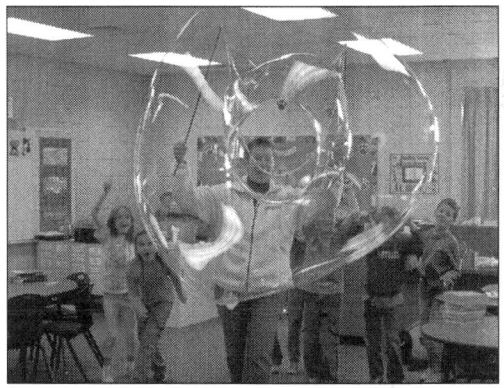

Laurie and her students enjoy creating the world's largest bubble!

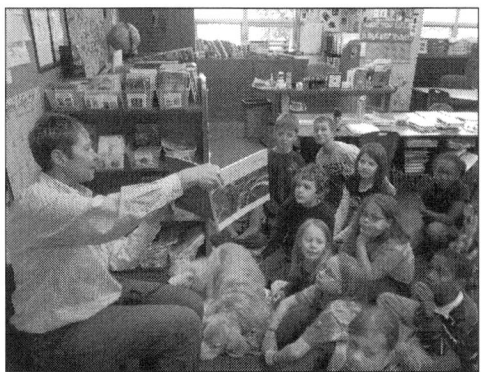

Laurie and Journey read to the kids.

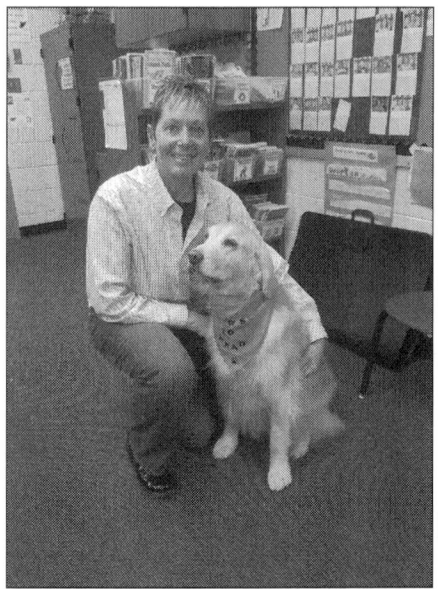

Laurie and Journey in the classroom.

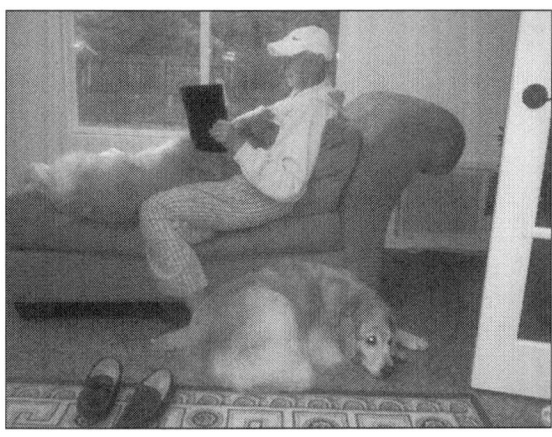

Laurie enjoying some golden love on a Sunday morning.

PART 3

Seeking Other Options

Not the News We Hoped For
October 30, 2012

We are back from our appointment, and unfortunately, we did not get the news we had hoped for. Certainly after our last PET scan, we were swinging for the deep seats. Unfortunately, as great as the fight has been from our champ, cancer gained a little ground this time.

Here's what we know. While the area in the lung is no longer a worry and the bones seem pretty darn good, the area in the breast grew a bit, and the liver continues to be an issue. One spot in the liver actually grew by one centimeter. When I look at a ruler, the optimist in me wants to say, "Well, one little centimeter is not that big a deal." And if I were measuring my foot or carpet or wallpaper, it wouldn't be. But growth of any kind when you're dealing with the enemy is not the direction you want to go.

We are back to figuring out the best way to knock this beast out of the park. The theory is that there is a cluster of cells within Laurie's liver that are resistant to the current chemo. That's the thing about cancer—it's wily and can learn to outfox the medicine. It appears that this has happened here—that while the chemo worked in many areas, it is not working in the liver. We need it to work in the liver. Period.

Dr. M. has recommended that we go to one of the leading breast cancer centers—MD Anderson in Texas. This will give us the benefit of hearing from another set of experts and a chance to possibly be part of a clinical trial. Clinical trials are on the cutting edge of treatment, and they may have one in their center that is tailor-made for Laurie. So we're waiting to hear on that appointment and will go from there.

As you can well imagine, our feet have been knocked out from under us. God is whispering to me to not forget all the good that has been done, and for that, I am so very thankful. The cancer is gone throughout most of Laurie's body. Thank goodness! I am just greedy enough to want it gone in all of Laurie's body.

She has fought so hard and has all the battle scars to prove it. I wanted her to have a break, to be able to rest easy and enjoy this beautiful world that she has created for all of us. I know very few things for sure, but I do know that this world is so much better, so much sweeter, so much kinder because Laurie Roth is in it. Please pray that God believes this too.

All Aboard!
November 3, 2012

As you can well imagine, it's been a rough week here in the Roth-Jones household. The news we received Tuesday was a shock that we did not anticipate. After all, we were riding the positive train. In our minds, we would only pull into beautiful, cancer-free stations, and there sure as heck would not be any derailments. In our minds, we would build upon the pretty route we had drawn up in August when all things cancer were moving in the right direction—out of Laurie's body. In our minds, Tuesday was the day when we would get off the cancer train and hopefully ride the positive train for the rest of our lives.

We were reminded Tuesday that this truly is a journey. The cancer train is a ride that we will probably never be completely off. And it will have hills and valleys, pretty scenery, and sometimes scary scenery. It will take us through dark tunnels that make us cry and over wide-open rails filled with sunshine. We would obviously prefer the days in the sun to the days in the dark. But as we have done all of our lives, we must buck up for the not-so-good days and bask in the wonderful ones. So far, we've been given so many more good days, and for that we are grateful.

I won't fool you. The superhero took a hit this week. And her typically optimistic sidekick, the one always able to put a positive spin on just about anything, was very nearly at a loss for words. After all, "the cancer in your liver has grown slightly" seems difficult to spin in an upbeat fashion. When you hear "it's gone up a notch" when it should have gone down, the applause stops dead in midclap. The words "there appear to be cells that are becoming resistant to the chemo" are the sucker punches of sucker punches. We wanted the cancer out, not growing. We wanted it cowering and begging for mercy, not standing stronger and growling. We wanted the cancer to fold like a house of cards, not build another neighborhood.

Yet there we were, hearing words that seemingly did not have any positive spin, any good side, anything to take our stomachs out of our throats. So we wallowed a bit. We walked around shocked and dismayed, sad and sadder depending on the day, the hour, or the minute. And for the very first time in our superhero's life, I think I briefly saw her knees give a bit. Not a full-on buckle, but they did dip. Why wouldn't they? Her cape had just been pulled by the meanest of bullies, and all of her weapons didn't seem enough to help her in the fight.

It was then that I felt that not-so-gentle nudge again. I'm telling you, it has to be my mother; the fingers are far too bony to be God's. Plus the words had a familiar ring. I had heard them many times before, in many conversations with my mom when she wanted me to buck up. In life, my mom always taught me to be brave and strong and step up to the plate. But in life, I always had her beside me, so being brave and strong made it easy to step up. After all, she'd catch me every time. Clearly, I've been hanging around superheroes all my life! And while one would think the superhero thing would rub off, I am safe in the role of trusty sidekick and secure in sometimes needing to be nudged.

So the nudge came, and the familiar words kept reminding me that I was only looking at the not-so-good stuff. This report didn't have the best news, but it was missing a lot of the bad news that we had gotten in May. The words that had previously sucker punched us five short months ago were not there. Why? Because the cancer wasn't there. The cancer wasn't in Laurie's spine, and it wasn't in her lung, and it wasn't in those upper lymph nodes. In fact, when we compare this report with the one in May, it is much shorter. Why? Because the cancer is gone in so many of the areas where it once was, so there is less to report. And that, dear army, deserves a big ol' AMEN!

But we can't ignore the big elephant in the room. As grateful as we are for the amazing results we have had, we are concerned that the cancer grew. While we were thinking it was exiting, it was actually slipping in the back door. We take solace in the words "slightly" and "a notch." And that's as far as it is going to go. We actually got a gift when cancer gave us this signal that it is on the move. Because guess what, cancer? We're on the move too, and we are faster! Well, Laurie is faster. Even with me on her coattails, she is faster, and she will win this race. Laurie is already gearing up for a bigger fight. I see it in her eyes, I hear it in her voice, I see the fire beginning to burn brighter in her belly. The champ may have gotten rocked, but it will be cancer that gets rolled—rolled right up and tossed out with the trash, where it belongs.

And along with you, our beautiful army, we are adding some new soldiers to the regime. We are adding the world-renowned MD Anderson Cancer Center to our ranks. If you go to their website, you will be amazed. You will see that the treatments they are doing are second to none and way ahead of the pack. You will see that their plans are not one size fits all, but tailor-made to the patient sitting in front of them. You will see that perhaps the reason we had to hear the news on Tuesday was to get MD Anderson in the fight.

Thank you for being with us all along this train ride, bumps and all. You have kept the train running this week with your cards and emails, texts and notes. You have spoiled us with your love, just like you have since we first pulled out of this crazy station. We're on the tracks again, this time headed to Texas. We've been contacted by their patient advocate center and will hear on Monday exactly when it is that we will go there. As soon as we know, you will know.

Your prayers and positive energy have always gotten us through! We know that you will be with us every mile of this ride. All aboard!

Deep in the Heart of Texas!
November 6, 2012

Well, Monday came and went, and despite my best efforts to pester, badger, and completely annoy our patient support advocate, Laydell, he was not to be budged. Laydell displayed the best customer service that I have ever seen as he sweetly put me off and distracted me with his calm demeanor and Texas accent. At one point, he even bet me that the review team's call would come in thirty minutes, and when it didn't and I tried to hold him to it, he had a smile in his voice and a sincere apology that the review team was not quite done. He told me that he knew the waiting was terrible and how sorry he was that we were going through this. Dang, Laydell was good! And I think he sensed that I was not the type to shoot the messenger.

But this morning, I awoke at 3:30 a.m. wishing I had his home number. We needed an appointment, and I could barely stand that we still did not have one. The clock ticked away, and soon it was 6:00 a.m. All I had to do was wait until 8:00, when Laydell would be just sitting down with his latte, ready to ease into his day, and then I would bombard his phone lines. Just as I was reaching for the phone, ours rang. Bless Laydell's heart. He was on the other end of the line with our appointment and all the specifics. Hearing his sweet, supportive voice made me overlook the fifty-two and a half hours it had taken him to make the appointment, not to mention the new gray hairs that had sprouted thanks to the wait.

Who am I kidding? The gray hairs would have come anyway, and Laydell just gave me someone to blame. The good news is that we have our appointment! On Monday, November 26 at 8:00 a.m., we will be meeting with Dr. A., a medical oncologist at MD Anderson. Judging by his credentials on the website, it sounds like he and Laurie are a match made in heaven. (Anyone surprised?) Dr. A. has done a lot of work in some of the areas that involve Laurie's type of breast cancer and is the guiding doctor on several clinical trials that could be appropriate for Laurie. No matter what, our champ will be seen by another world-renowned expert who will review her case and her treatment and chart a course for her success. I'm in love with Dr. A. already!

Laurie's Journey

So off we go to Texas. This Chicago girl doesn't stand a chance. A few of Laydell's phrases made me reach for my Texan-to-English dictionary that dear friends and neighbors dropped off for us this weekend. My hope is that no matter how the doctors say it, whether it be in Texan, Chicagoan, or Central Illinoisan, they say, "We got this!" When I hear that, who knows what could happen. I may just do the "Boot Scootin' Boogie"!

While we will be deep in the heart of Texas, each of you will be deep in our hearts. Your support and love and unwavering belief that we will win this fight has often been the difference maker for both of us. That's not changing now. To hear your sweet words of nothing but full-on support as we navigate our little bump in the road is truly what sustains both Laurie and me. When our hearts went dark, you turned the lights back on. When our eyes filled with fearful tears, your hands reached out to dry them. When the weight of worry just seemed too much, you helped carry the load. God gave each of you to us as the most perfect of presents, the most awesome of armies, the most loving of lifesavers. And to you and to God, we say Amen.

Our champ is hanging in there. She's anxious to get back in the fight, because she has so much to live for. But she remembers the fight all too well—the fight that took her nails, that beat her up and loved off all her hair. Our champ has her dukes up and her chin up, and she is oh so ready to punch the lights out of cancer. Who is this superhero? I'll tell you who: she is the great Laurie Roth that God made, God knows, and God remembers. And I believe that when all is said and done, God will reward her with more good days than not-so-good, more healthy days than crappy ones, all surrounded by the best army of family and friends ever assembled. The one downside will be her darn sidekick. The Chicago accent has been hard enough for Laurie to bear; imagine when the sidekick comes on home with a Texas one! Yee-hah, y'all! And in Texan that means "AMEN!"

Amazing Grace
November 22, 2012

Today we celebrate Thanksgiving. If tradition holds true, I will overeat, I will complain about overeating, and then I will overeat again approximately four hours later. What I will also do is give thanks. I will humbly reflect upon all the gifts that I have been given, not just over this year, but throughout my life. I will give thanks for my wonderful family, both on earth and in heaven, and my extended family made up of each of you. And I will give thanks to God for allowing me to be Laurie's sidekick. There are many gifts for which I have bowed my head, closed my eyes, and whispered words of humble thanks. But the gift of sharing the road with Laurie is one for which I am so very thankful.

I have frequently called Laurie "grace under fire." You've heard me, you're read it in these pages, you'll read it again. Many days, she is "Amazing Grace." But on any given day of the week, she is simply but perfectly, "Grace." Why? Take a peek in the dictionary and you'll understand. The dictionary defines grace as "God's favor." I told you that you'd get it. I'm smiling too. Is that not perfect? If you know Laurie, if you have shared even one minute with her, you get the distinct feeling that God showed you *favor* by placing you beside His *favorite*. I like to think of Laurie as his favor to me. Having said that, please know that I know that God sure didn't owe me any favors. Nope, not even one. I've been pulling in favors from God for years, so I'm actually the one who owes Him big-time! Yet here I am, owed absolutely nothing, sharing my life with a person who helps complete it. How ridiculously crazy is that? If that's not amazing grace, then I don't know what is.

Beyond being one of the biggest favors ever done for me, Laurie gives me a shining example every day of how to do this thing called life. Throughout this journey, if I'd had my druthers, there would have been many a day when I would have stayed in bed, getting up only long enough to roll around on the floor wailing or, at most, mustering the energy to throw one pity party after another. On the best of my worst days, I'd probably do a combination of all three. I'd fill my hours with "uh-ohs", throw in a few mutterings of "Hadn't thought of that scary idea before," and plenty of my go-to thought as I enter my downward descent, the ever-dreaded "What if . . ." The "what ifs" will get you every time. They're infinitely unanswerable and can keep your mind spinning for hours. Trust me, I've timed them. I know this all too well.

Fortunately, I share my life with someone who doesn't go down What If Road, and she sure doesn't spend any time on Poor Me Lane. In fact, her favorite route is to take It Could Be So Much Worse Street straight over to I Bet Tomorrow Will Be Better Court. Dang that Laurie—I'm trying to wallow, and she's heck-bent on making me thankful. I live with the epitome of Thanksgiving every single day!

That is not to say that this angel on earth doesn't sometimes start to feel the weight of her wings. She does. Her wings have had to carry a lot, especially these last four months. They've felt the weight of chemo and its nasty side effects, of tough tests and tougher results, of dark days and long nights. She has worried at times and cried at others. She has wondered how much she can take, and then she has gotten up and taken some more. She's seen hell on earth and yet leans on heaven.

Through it all, she remains thankful. Thankful that it's not worse. Thankful that most of the beast is gone. Thankful for being able to go to MD Anderson and meet with the experts who train the experts. Through this entire fight, her wings may have gotten a little bent and her body pretty bruised, but her spirit is very much intact. Through it all, her smile is as pretty as ever and her laugh still the best sound that I have ever heard. Through it all, she has stood firm and strong, always reminding me that we will win this. I've never doubted a single word she's ever uttered, and I'm not about to start now. My money has been, and always will be, on God's favor. Amen.

So today, while saying grace, define yours. I bet God has also shown you a favor or two. I bet that you have one of God's favors, or many favors, sitting right next to you, or at the very least, there with you in spirit. I know we do. Whether you are right beside us or with us in spirit, how very thankful we are for you. You have been our army, our lifesavers, and throughout this journey, you have certainly been our favors. Happy Thanksgiving!

Making Cancer History!
November 27, 2012

Yesterday was a day of doctors' visits and pokes and prodding of our champ. We met Dr. A. and his team, who are now OUR team. They all had reviewed Laurie's records, knew them by heart, had bookmarked important dates and results, and recited them to us. They examined Laurie, asked additional questions, and made us feel as though in this sea of thousands of people, we were their only concern. They have taken "personalized medicine" to new heights. And when they were done, Dr. A. looked at Laurie, with her hair still loved off but coming back, with her fingernails still playing hide-and-seek and her pretty smile still intact, and said what we had been holding our breath to hear.

He said, "We have so many options for you." Options equal hope. Hope equals future. Future equals yippee-yi-yay! Yes, it's official. I am now speaking cowpoke. However, Laurie has limited, almost banned, my use of the term "y'all." Apparently I used it too many times on the drive to Chicago. It is just like me to blow my wad of "y'alls" before we even touched the ground of Texas!

Here's what we have on tap for the week: more tests, more scans, biopsies, and more conferences with the team. While Laurie has already had these tests and scans done, the experts who train the experts want their own. They take the labs and the tissue and examine them in nitty-gritty detail. And when they know each and every protein and the molecular makeup of each and every tiny cell, they will present us with a tailor-made targeted therapy regimen just for Laurie Roth. Is there anyone more deserving of such a personalized gift? I don't think so!

Our superhero has her cape back on and ready to go. It's a little torn, a little tattered, but our girl has it on and she is ready to fight. Cape on. Gloves on. GAME ON! We love MD Anderson's motto: "Making Cancer History." Isn't that awesome? And that's exactly what Dr. A. and the team are aiming to do for Laurie—make her cancer history! Amen!

And by the way, it is true that everything really is bigger in Texas. Your great love and support sure are! We feel them every minute of every day. You send your prayers and your positive energy, and we are buoyed by your love. The comfort that you send is HUGE! Thank you so much.

Testing 1-2-3
November 29, 2012

I think we're going to have to start calling our champ by a new name: "Pincushion" is more like how she is feeling. Maybe we could change it temporarily to Champion Pincushion. Because despite how many times she is stuck with a needle for this test and that test, she smiles, laughs with the techs, and takes it all in stride. She is an absolute champ as she keeps taking one after another for the team.

We've had three straight days of tests. MD Anderson is extremely thorough, leaving no stone unturned as they search through Laurie's entire body to find all the clues that cancer has left. Then they will compile all the information and put together the tailor-made treatment plan that I mentioned in my last post. It will be specific to Laurie and include not just one option, but numerous backup options as well. It was music to our ears when Dr. A. said that along with plan A, he would "also be putting together a plan B and plan C and so on." Again, that beautiful word: options. Options give us great hope. Hope leads to our great future. Our future leads to me getting to say "yippee-yi-yay" every single day!

I'm keeping those to myself right now, because my inner cowpoke is outwardly annoying. I need to be a more quiet cheerleader and trusty sidekick and save my "yee-hahs" and "y'alls" for another time. Today is going to be a tough one for our girl. She's already been injected once with dye and just finished a bone scan. In an hour, we'll go back and they'll inject her with another type of dye. We'll wait a couple of hours for that to move through her body, and then she'll have CT scans. Our girl has done a lot of heavy lifting this week, all with a beautiful smile and fighter's spirit.

Laurie's Journey

My eyes fill up as I reflect that no matter what Laurie has to go through as we race toward our cure, she does so with the most beautiful and gentle spirit. She does so with a quiet commitment that she'll not just win this race, but run with arms held high in victory. Every day she gives me another reason to declare her not just my hero, but my superhero. These past four days have been no exception. Her fighting spirit always arrives to take the next test, be poked, and be prodded. But it is her amazing grace, her inner and outer beauty, and her gentle spirit that bring peace to all of us standing in her shadow. People are as drawn to her in these rooms in Houston as they are in the chemo room back home. They are warmed by her smile, they love to hear her laugh, and they soak up that beautiful spirit that is pure Laurie Roth. And pure Laurie Roth will be the reason we will win! Amen.

We have done some fun stuff too—we have shopped, we have eaten, and we have laughed. Laurie and I laugh a lot, firmly believing it is one of the best medicines around. I marvel that no matter what she's been through, she can still laugh. Along with laughing, we've walked our feet off. MD Anderson is a huge facility, so you walk a lot while you're here. There are expanded golf cart shuttles that will take you from one end to the other, but I feel too guilty to get on when Laurie is insistent on walking—darn her and her exercise gene! But I do look longingly each time a shuttle whizzes past us. So we've laughed, we've walked, and we've met amazing people. As Laurie quickly reminds me, there are people so much worse. And while I believe that we are entitled to take some time to think and pray about our worst, I am thankful that we have this worst and nothing more.

We will be returning tomorrow to Illinois. They haven't been able to get all of our tests done, so another trip back is in our immediate future, probably in about two weeks or less. Laurie does need to have another liver biopsy, and unfortunately, that couldn't be booked while we were here. Hurry up and wait is our new mantra. But wait we will, and return we will, so that we can get our plan A and plan B and plan C. We will return to get our future.

With your prayers, God's hands, and Laurie's spirit, we are looking forward to our future. And y'all are a huge part of that! This is the best army ever. Thank you for being here with us in spirit—we love each of you and are thankful that you are in our lives.

Home Again, Home Again, Jiggity Jig!
December 1, 2012

Laurie's reading the paper, so this ol' cowpoke has the run of the computer! If she can't hear me, then my inner Texan can come out big-time (or "big-tom," as we say in Houston)! I learned that it's not "smiling," it's "smalling," and when we were "tired," we were actually "tarred." Who knew? And if you're wondering who "Heidi" is, that's actually Texan for "howdy"! It took me two full days to figure out who in the world Heidi was every time we got a good ol' Texas hello. I got a lot more time in my day after I could stop looking over my shoulder for Heidi.

It is so good to be home. Home with our four-legged babies; home, where we longed to be the whole time we were gone; home, glorious home. If you haven't figured it out, Laurie and I don't venture far from home. We've built a good one, enjoy our pets completely, and if we leave home, we rarely leave without them. In short, we're freaks. We know it, and we're just fine with it. No counseling required! At least not for that aspect.

Laurie's Journey

Our arrival home was just what we knew it would be: a reunion of the best kind! Journey and Harbour were right at the door the second they heard our car pull in. Hobo was right behind them. And to everyone's surprise, so was Alicat. Ali primarily remains on her throne and lets her minions come to her. Apparently, she actually missed her loyal subjects, so she graced them with a wonderful welcome, even allowing herself to be picked up! It's so much easier to be adored when you are being held by one of your minions.

The reunion went on for quite some time: Journey running around, picking up various toys and romping around the house with them; Harbour rubbing herself into us as if she couldn't get close enough, all the while squealing with complete delight. Who am I kidding? We were all squealing in delight. It was just what our weary bones and tired spirits needed—pure four-legged love!

I have written about the love and comfort that Laurie gets from these wonderful nurses of ours. On days that knocked hard on the champ, it was these four that made her get up, get going, get living. It was the faces of these four pets looking adoringly at her, knowing what I have known for so long: that Laurie truly hangs the moon. It was their perfectly placed paws on Laurie's so very weary bones that gave her the will to stand up and stand strong to face the day. It was these little spirits carrying hers when the champ's arms were just a bit too tired to do it for herself. What she could always do, no matter what, was do anything for them.

So this past week was hard without our four-legged Florence Nightingales. I tried to fill the void. But how do you fill up the space that is always perfectly covered with Journey, Harbour, Ali, and Hobo? I can make Laurie laugh. I can be beside her for every test and every scan, wishing that I could take the needle pricks and prodding probes for her. I can tie her superhero cape up close to her chin, smile a confident smile, and remind her that *nobody* saves our world like she does. But the truth of the matter is, these little spirits come perfectly packaged with just the right medicine that is needed at just the right time. And now that we're home, we're practically overdosing on their love!

A big thank-you goes out to the angels who cared for our pals while we were gone. We had many offers, and we felt so blessed that people were so willing to take care of the pets. Thank you to all of you who asked, thought about them, and thought about us while we were apart.

Journey and Harbour were lovingly and perfectly cared for in the home of our dear friends, Sue and Al. They were exercised, they were played with, and most important, they were loved. When I leave this world, I want to return as a dog in the house of Sue and Al! It truly is dog heaven right here on earth. And it is clear that Journey and Harbour found that out too. Thank you, Sue and Al!

Hobo and Alicat were cared for by a team of people to whom big thanks go out. Our neighbor Vicki came by early in the morning and then later at night to check on them. Our dear friend Kris, from whom we originally got Ali, came and played with Hobo and was actually allowed to pet Queen Ali. Apparently, Ali does remember her roots and appreciates from whence she came. Our wonderful friends Lisa and Lisa also came by and checked on the felines. Ali actually likes them and allows them to grace her presence, and sometimes she even rewards Lisa M. by sitting on her lap. This week was no exception. By all of his caretakers, Hobo was found to be the rodeo clown that I have described. Look for him and his antics to soon be part of a YouTube sensation! In so many ways, it's like the ghost of our dear Max Jones is back in the house! This Hobo boy never fails to entertain!

Along with the relief that our babies were as well cared for as if we were with them, we had your texts, your calls, your emails, and sweet, sweet posts and "likes" on our blog. We had your prayers and your positive thoughts carrying our spirits. We had you tucked in the very corners of our hearts, and we would pull from you the strength and the comfort that we so often and sometimes desperately needed to face the day, face the night, face the world. Thank you one and all!

On the Road Again
December 8, 2012

Just a quick update to let you know that we take off for good ol' Houston tomorrow. Our return will be on Thursday. We are praying that our travel path involves the use of only our car and their airplanes. We are just fine with skipping the bus and the train that we had to use the last go-round. In this case, less really is more.

At this time, we know that Laurie will have a liver biopsy and an ultrasound, meet with a pain management doctor, and then meet with our guy, Dr. A. Of all the things that she will be put through, aside from traveling with me, the liver biopsy will be, by far, the worst. She's had one of these before and clearly remembers it as something that she would never put on her "must do again" list. But being the trouper that she is, she knows that this is an essential test to get us to the finish line. She knows that she has to go through this not-one-bit-fun procedure so that the most precise treatment plan can be put in place. She knows that she has to go through the rain to get to the sunshine—again.

That's been a frequent refrain in our house—we walk in the dark a bit to get to the light. Standing in Laurie's shadow, I'm very lucky to get to see light every day. I see it in her smile, in her laugh, in her amazing ability to get out of bed when it would be so much easier to pull the covers up over her head and say "uncle" to the upcoming day. I think we all know that this is more my mode than Laurie's. In fact, if I had my preference, I'd be typing this from bed. But Laurie? No way. She's up and at 'em, ready to go and greet the day. She isn't wasting one minute of this life—and that, my friends, is why she holds the keys to the kingdom in this fight.

It is for this very reason that she will be in the winner's circle and cancer will be doing the walk of shame (as well it should, for messing not once with sweet Laurie Roth, but twice!). It is for this very reason that Laurie will be victorious, hands over head, breaking the tape at the finish line. And it is for this very reason that when all of this beautiful vision becomes reality, this wonderful army will be able to do a jump for joy, say a "yahooey Louie," and in homage to our team in Texas, a "yee-hah, y'all!"

The suitcases are getting packed with all the essentials: clothes, toiletries, Texan-to-English dictionary, my newly acquired southern drawl that Laurie made me leave with Security on departure, lots of pictures of our furry buddies, and your positive and loving spirits. With that, I think the checklist of travel items is complete! Though "we" are working on paring back the number of shoes that were brought for the last trip. Not sure if you know this, but I live with the Imelda Marcos of America. So in true Imelda fashion, one carry-on bag was entirely devoted to Laurie's shoe selection. I had two pairs: loafers and slippers (since my anal-retentive personality will not allow my bare feet to touch the floor of a hotel room). Meanwhile, Laurie's shoe side of the room looked like the shoe department at Von Maur. I was waiting for one of the cleaning staff to ask if we had something in a size 7. Anyway, traveling light is not our strong suit, but standing strong is Laurie's signature move, and for that she needs good shoes, and so she shall have them!

Having said that, please keep our champ in your prayers and positive thoughts. God built her not to break, but her shoulders are getting tired of the wait. It is the waiting that can exhaust you. But I know our superhero. All she needs are the results, a treatment plan, her four-legged nursemaids, all of you, and this trusty ol' sidekick, and she will be kicking tail and taking names! I know you're thinking that I channeled my inner cowpoke for that last saying, but unfortunately, I've been saying that one all on my own for far too many years. Again, not a proud statement, but a true one.

And another true statement is that your love and support have poured in this week and bolstered the weary hearts of two tired travelers. Your cards have been awesome, and your well-timed calls, emails, and texts were absolute spirit lifters. We felt the power of your prayers and your positive thoughts just when we needed them the most. You are with us every step of the way, and for that we will always be thankful.

When You Wish Upon a Star
December 13, 2012

The champ and her cowpoke are back from the Lone Star State! We were on the go the entire trip. If Laurie wasn't getting poked, prodded, biopsied, or examined by someone, then we were waiting for her to be poked, prodded, biopsied, or examined by someone. It was a jam-packed four days, as we suspected it would be. But we are home now, surrounded by golden retriever love, Hobo hugs, and Alicat dirty looks. Ah. All's right with the world!

First the news regarding Laurie's scans: we have some victories to report! The bone scan is primarily clear! From the top of her beautiful head to the bottom of her baby toes, Laurie's bone scan looked very good. There is one little spot on her fourth rib, but that is connected to the growth in her breast. Hooray for the champ! The lungs look perfect. No cancer seen in either lung! Nicely done, superhero! Her heart was also scanned and, as we all know, it is perfect. Considering all of the chemo that she has had over the past four years, and knowing that chemo can do quite a number on the ol' ticker, Laurie's is perfect. As if any of us had any doubt how that was going to read. So to recap: bones—great, lungs—excellent, heart—perfect! Those are all in the win column for our girl, and she richly deserves a big round of applause.

As we knew before we even boot-scooted into Texas, the liver and breast had actually progressed at some point during the last three rounds of chemo. So we weren't surprised to find out that the scans still showed tumor activity. The good news is that it isn't taking over either area. In fact, Dr. A. explained that the cancer is occupying about 10 to 15 percent of her liver. While this isn't a stunning amount to an oncologist, these are tenants that you don't want. What you want is for them to be shown the door—and not in a polite way. Same for the growth in the breast—freeloading time is over! It may be only 8 millimeters, but that's too much space and it's time for it to be escorted out.

To that end, we are bringing in some new bodyguards in the form of a three-drug combo. The acronym for this heavyweight is FEC, with each letter standing for a different chemo agent. Dr. A. said that the FEC cocktail was actually created by two MD Anderson scientists years ago. It is now the go-to combo used across the world for handling noisy squatters like Laurie's. This place is absolutely amazing!

We went to MD Anderson because Dr. M. felt that we were at a crossroads for treatment. He knew that Laurie's cancer had grown wise to his weapons. He made the excellent recommendation that we go to the experts who train the experts and get them to tell us what our next move should be against this beast. I wish I had a picture of Dr. A.'s smile when he said, "Miss Roth, I want you to go on FEC. It is the gold standard of treatment!" With his wonderful accent, his kind eyes, and his warm smile, he reminded both of us that we were right where we needed to be, that we had added amazing teammates to the roster, and that we were in such good hands.

While we are so thankful that the tests support good news, we are mindful that the road is long, especially for our girl. The FEC will be administered once every three weeks. Laurie will do that for three rounds (nine weeks), and then we will go back to Texas to be scanned. We have faith that the gold standard will do the trick, but our champ's shoulders are not going to get a break. FEC will not be easy. It will love off the hair that started coming back, it may make any nail that dared to grow again start to head south, and on the worst days, it will make our girl wonder which is worse: the treatment or the cancer. As her trusty sidekick, I will remind her that the treatment is temporary, cancer will absolutely be temporary, but the life she leads is a permanent gift to all of us. Her life is certainly permanently etched on my heart, and I am privileged to stand beside this superhero. It is Laurie's beautiful life that reminds all of us that even on the darkest nights, you can often find a shining star.

Tonight is actually one of those nights. Nerd alert! Nerd alert! I'm about to go all Cliff Clavin from *Cheers* on you—there is a meteor shower that will start tonight and is slated to be the year's best. It will go through tomorrow night, with over one hundred meteors, a.k.a. shooting stars, being visible every hour. Can you believe the timing? We return from Texas with a new game plan in hand and three new, really mean fighters all ready to team up with the champ and beat the beast into oblivion, and the heavens are opening up with a glorious light show! We are being given not just a little ol' bright night, but a shower of shooting stars for the next twenty-four hours. It's like God and all of His angels are winking at us!

I don't know about you, but when I see a shooting star racing across the sky, I make a wish. I'm getting my coat on, bundling up, and heading outside. I have a bootful of Texas wishes, all asking for my heart's desire and my one dream to come true: that Laurie wins! Tonight, please make this your wish too.

FEC Means "Fully Eliminating Cancer"
December 20, 2012

We met with Dr. M. yesterday and went over all of the results from the Texas tests, as well as the new game plan of FEC. Laurie will start this regimen on Thursday, December 27. We all agreed that the champ had earned her holiday and could certainly wait to start the toxins until after Christmas. Whew!

Laurie's Journey

We've been looking at this waiting period as Laurie's bulk-up time. I've been trying to get her to eat whatever she wants to eat, enjoy what she wants to enjoy, and do whatever her little ol' heart desires. This has meant taking Journey and Harbour on long walks in all sorts of fun spots around town. It has meant that the house is decorated to the nines and may actually be rivaling the Griswold's from *Christmas Vacation*. And of course, it has meant that I've had to take more walks, exercise my very out-of-shape heart, and put out more energy in the great outdoors than I ever really intended. What's next? Vacuuming? How much can one person take?

We know a little about this FEC regimen. We know that it will bring a lot of the old side effects that we saw in the previous regimen. We know that Laurie will feel pretty puny for at least five to seven days, will be highly vulnerable to infection, and will not have much of an appetite. We also know that her hair and nails will more than likely not stick around too long. Those of you who have seen Laurie recently know that her nails showed back up and her hair was coming in quite nicely. If you've watched her in action, you know that the Energizer Bunny has been whipping around with more energy than a roomful of toddlers. If you know her, you know that when given the opportunity, Laurie Roth chooses to live life every second of every day.

And therein lies the rub. Our champ is at the top of her game right now—feeling good, feeling fine, feeling sassy! It's hard to believe by looking at her that in one week she will have to walk through the doors of the cancer center, get poked, get prodded, and get chemo. She will have to be sick to be better. She will have to be brave to not be scared. She will have to fight to win so as not to lose even one inch to this mean, nasty beast. As you well know,

Laurie Roth doesn't do sick, she doesn't do scared, and she sure doesn't do losing! As hard as it is to move from feeling so darn good today to feeling so darn crummy in a week, she will do it, because that is what a superhero does. She puts on her cape, she makes evil obey, and in doing so, she saves the world every single day. From the bottom of my grateful heart, thank you, superhero.

So the twenty-seventh is the day that FEC takes the beast on. As our dear friend Judith posted, FEC is our new favorite acronym. It may mean three really long medical terms, but in Judith's words, it now means "fully eliminating cancer"! Yippee-yi-yay yahoo! Oh, by the way, Laurie is allowing a few Texas terms and a Chicago-style southern drawl to pepper my vocabulary. As you can imagine, I am giddy with the latitude! I actually think she secretly likes it—or it's a Christmas miracle! Regardless, I say a big ol' yee-hah, y'all!

We also say a big ol' thank-you for all of your love and support. Your prayers and thoughts bring comfort that only this group of lifesavers could deliver. You remind us every single day that we are not alone, that we are loved, and that we will win. And to that, we say AMEN!

We Wish You a Merry Christmas
December 25, 2012

As we begin the various celebrations of this day, Laurie and I wanted to wish all of our beautiful army of lifesavers a very Merry Christmas! Of all the gifts that we will open, we will always be most thankful for the gift of you. At some point in life's journey, you came beautifully packaged in pretty paper, pretty ribbon, pretty bows. We knew when we met you that we were opening gifts not just for the moment, but for the long run. We knew we had gifts that would span a lifetime. We had gifts that would become our lifelines.

On dark, silent nights when we could find little joy in our world, you reminded us that there would be peace on earth. You helped us hear God's voice as he beckoned all his faithful, joyful and triumphant. We found ourselves on dark streets shining with the everlasting light, allowing our hopes and fears of all our years to be met with God's perfect love. It was your love that helped these two weary souls find reason to rejoice and enjoy the new and beautiful morn that was about to break. You gave us the strength to dream by the fire, to face unafraid all the plans that we've made, and to walk through a winter wonderland. You are faithful friends who are dear to us, who gather near to us, and in doing so, you make all our troubles seem miles away.

You knew that we would need a little music, need a little laughter, need a little singing, ringing through the rafter. Heaven knows that I pray every day for a happy ever after. Like little angels sitting on our shoulders, you know that we need a little Christmas, often right this very minute, and you never fail to deliver. You truly are the wonderful things that we remember all through our lives. While I usually want a hippopotamus for Christmas, and only a hippopotamus will do, this year may our day most simply, and most perfectly, be merry and bright. And you know what? As I listen to Laurie laugh and feel both of us being warmed by the love of our wonderful pets and thoughts of each of you, it truly is shaping up to be the most wonderful time of the year.

Although it's been said, many times, many ways, from the bottom of our hearts, Merry Christmas to you.

What Lies Within Us
December 27, 2012

You may have heard the saying "What lies behind us and what lies before us are tiny matters compared to what lies within us."

We all know what is now behind Laurie. We're all up to speed as to what lies before her. And try as I might to detail what lies within her, I don't know that I will ever properly capture the strength and toughness that is our very own superhero. What I do know is that what lies within her is what has and always will be the difference maker in this fight.

Cancer knows one way to act: mean. Laurie doesn't do mean. She couldn't be mean if you paid her. Trust me, I've challenged her enough with my antics that "mean" would have showed up a long time ago if she had it in her. But cancer may have thought that Laurie's sweetness and kindness meant that she's not a fighter. Oh, cancer, you silly, silly demon. Within Laurie Roth lies a fighter of the greatest kind. Hits that knock most people to their knees barely make her flinch. Sucker punches below the belt may sting, but she will never let you see her sweat. And just when her foe thinks she's on the ropes, she tucks her head, focuses inward, and comes out swinging! Pink boxing gloves make the victory all the sweeter (and prettier, quite frankly).

So today started another round in this match. This cancer hasn't really seen the likes of the combination it received today. The FEC crew has some new drugs that Laurie's cancer doesn't know about. In fact, one is actually called the Red Devil. I'm not making that up. What better way to fight the demon but with another one! The sneak attack on cancer is usually your best bet. If you catch it off guard with new weapons, it doesn't have time to figure out your game plan. So that's what we're doing—hitting it hard with FEC and then punching it again with Laurie's amazing fighting spirit. This is the perfect combo! FEC will tear through Laurie's body looking for each and every little cancer cell. It will find one, punch its lights out, and then move on to the next one. When it has whipped through Laurie's entire body, it will start right back again, combing every nook and cranny for the beast that hides within her.

Then what lies within Laurie's spirit, within her heart, within that beautiful soul of hers will do the rest. When most would raise the white flag in surrender, Laurie stands stronger, ready for more fight. She gets up when her body says "stay down." She walks the dogs when her bones are aching and her feet hurting. She will live this wonderful life that she has been given, ignoring the monster banging on the door. Laurie Roth doesn't quit, and today was no exception.

We have taken long walks into the cancer center before, but none as long as today's seemed to be. Even with a close parking spot, it took us both a very long time to walk through those doors. More than any other day, we were reminded that this journey is a marathon, and somehow it just added another mile. Walking in, watching her put her game face on, seeing her take her fears and put them to the side, made a lump form in my throat and my eyes well up with tears. Knowing that Laurie was doing the exact thing that we had prayed so hard to put behind her, knowing that what lies in front of her is no walk in the park, my heart broke in two for her. So much so that I kind of lost sight of what lies within her.

I almost forgot who we are dealing with. It's Laurie Roth, superhero, champion, victor. Does she want to be all those things? No. But she knows she has to. She is the one who will always do what has to be done. The very act that she didn't think she could muster up the strength to do, she did. The very thing that was the number one thing she never wanted to do again, she knew she had to do. The very thought of more chemo making her more sick was almost enough to make her run the other way. I said "almost," folks. Because what lies within Laurie is the desire to do what absolutely has to be done. Whether it is the right thing for family, for friends, for the fight of her life, she will always, always do it. And that, dear army, is the difference maker. God built her not to break, and he sure built her not to give in. Amen.

So in she walked, accompanied by me, her trusty sidekick, and the added bonus of her little sister Jenny. Like Laurie, Jenny has a smile that lights up a room, so the chemo room got a big ol' dose of Roth sunshine. It was just what the doctor ordered for all of us and everyone who basked in the light of their smiles. The cinnamon rolls Jenny was carrying didn't hurt either!

Laurie made conversation with those around her, making their chemo time go faster and easier. She talked to a retired carpenter and listened so patiently and intently as he described all the items he can make from scraps of countertops. His wife was acting engrossed in the May 2009 issue of *Good Housekeeping*, and I had begun to count the ceiling tiles, but Laurie, she listened. When the carpenter left, she talked to another guy, named Chauncey, who is fighting bone cancer. They talked about their chemo, their side effects, their dogs, and their lives. Chauncey talked so much he ended up telling Laurie, "I'm really a pretty quiet guy, but somehow I've talked more to you than I have anyone in a long time." Yep, Chauncey, she has that effect on people. You talk, she listens. She listens, you feel better. You feel better, she feels better. Win-win. That's how it works in Laurie's world.

Laurie's Journey

She will do what she has to do to get to the win for everyone. She listens, she cares, she loves. And when she does all of these things, she lives. She lives exactly how she thinks it works best: to do for others, to do the right thing, to do what she has to do. Ol' Chauncey got a glimpse of our superhero's cape as she took care of his universe, if only for the four hours they shared together.

But the cape may get a little tattered this go-round. For the short term, we know that the next five days will be hard on her. Today and tomorrow will be no walk in the park, but they will probably pale in comparison to the side effects of days three through five. While this treatment is supposed to be a bit better tolerated than the last one, it's still chemo, and it has quite a kick. We hope that after that, life will begin to be okay. It won't be normal, but we'll take okay. Since these are new fighters, led by one called the Red Devil, who knows. What I do know is that Laurie's spirit is amazing, her heart strong and focused, and her laugh still one of the best sounds heaven ever gave me. May I hear her laugh soon; may I hear her laugh more; may I always, always hear her laugh.

Please keep her in your hearts and in your prayers. This is the marathon for which we had already unlaced our shoes. (Who am I kidding? I never even put my shoes on, let alone laced them up, preferring to be in the pace car.) So getting back into the race is a tough one mentally and certainly a tough one physically for anyone, even our girl. She will need the collective love of all God's people, just like you have given us every step of the way. Thank you for your love, your constant care, your unfailing support that helps us through the long, dark stretches. You are lifesavers of the highest order! We love each and every one of you.

Whose Side Are You On, FEC?
December 30, 2012

It's been a rough weekend so far, with the side effects rolling in like Sherman tanks, one after the other. First to arrive were flulike symptoms. And not just your run-of-the-mill flu, though that would be bad enough. This is the flu multiplied by a thousand. It's like the flu bug invited all of its ugly, nasty, and very exhausting relatives—the loud ones, the ones that eat all your food and always, always sit in your favorite chair. *Those* relatives. Laurie's skin hurt, her bones ached, her joints were so very sore. Just to shower and get dressed pretty much took the wind out of our girl's sails.

Then, as if that wasn't enough, in came the mouth and tongue sores. Those arrived in the middle of the night, like impolite houseguests that think it's okay to wake you up at two in the morning just to let you know that they're going to stay for another couple of days. Greeeeat. Of course, these are not just your ordinary mouth sores, either, nor do they really even compare to a fever blister or cold sore. Unless you have had fifty-three cold sores or blisters all over your mouth and tongue at once. Then it's exactly like what Laurie has. While she is making herself eat some soup and making herself keep the fluids up, talking is at a minimum because it's just too painful.

The funny thing about this journey is that even though you have a feeling about what is coming down the pike for you, even though you've seen your share of side effects and can try to prepare, you never really know for sure how your body is going to react until the side effects take effect. And then you don't really know to what degree they are going to happen until they do. Laurie and I lead orderly lives, lives that are not left to chance, and surprises aren't really our strong suit. So we have had to really try to be flexible and be ready for whatever gets thrown our way. Mouth sores? We've got a medicated rinse for that. It doesn't work that well, but we have it. Painful skin? We have the lightest of fabrics washed and ready to wear, and still Laurie's skin will hurt if anything touches it or bumps it. Body aches? We have five hundred Tylenol capsules sitting in the medicine cabinet—and they won't probably touch the pain and discomfort that this battle brings. But we're ready!

It's par for the course, just the way this fight is fought, the way you have to get through it. The only way through it is, well, through it. And the only way I know how to help is to remind Laurie all the time that nobody does it better. Despite how poorly she is feeling, she maintains our normalcy, our security, our life. When her body aches and her skin hurts and her head pounds, she looks at me and says, "I am not going to waste this day." That is code for "Get your shoes on, we're taking the dogs for a walk." When her mouth fills with blisters and she manages to croak out "I have to keep eating so I can continue with my medicine," that means we're making a soup or two and I need to get the cutting boards out so we can get chopping. And when it almost seems too much and the champ appears to be on the ropes, she will look at me and say, "I can do this, right?" That is my signal that this sidekick needs to buck up and remind her superhero that she is unbeatable, unstoppable, absolutely and completely unbelievable with the strength she delivers to this fight!

FEC's strength can make us wonder whose side it actually is on. It's like a Pac-Man game completely out of control—eating the bad cells and, clearly, devouring the good ones too. It is in the fight with us, and for that we are thankful, but maybe it needs to back off the steroids! With it in the ring, it's more like Rock 'Em Sock 'Em Robots! It has a one-two punch that Ali would appreciate. Right now we're seeing the impact of those punches on Laurie. And I am on my hands and knees praying that in nine weeks, the scans at MD Anderson will see the impact of those punches on the cancer cells. In fact, they can Rock 'Em Sock 'Em to the next planet! Then that will be code for CELEBRATION!

Please keep Laurie in your prayers, and keep sending your positive energy. While she is as tough as they come, these are trying days, and strength in the valleys is as important, and possibly more important, than strength on the mountaintops. May these side effects go as quickly as they came so that Laurie can do what she does so well: LIVE!

Go Out and Do Good
January 1, 2013

Go into the world and do well. But more importantly, go into the world and do good.
—Dr. Minor Myers Jr., seventeenth president of Illinois Wesleyan University

In the fourteen years that he was president of the university, Dr. Myers closed each and every graduation ceremony at Wesleyan with the above words. I remember reading those words in a newspaper article about Dr. Myers. They resonated in me, they impacted me, and they stuck. Not that I thought, "Hey, that's me! I run around doing good for others all the time!" No. Unfortunately, no. They stuck and gave me something better to shoot for. I had these words hanging in my office for years. Every day I try to meet the goal of doing good. Some days I do better than others. Some days I succeed, some days I don't. But I give it a shot.

I live with someone who not only gives these words a shot, but succeeds every single day in doing well and doing good. Although we live just a mile or so from Wesleyan, to my knowledge, Laurie and Dr. Myers never met. But I will tell you, every time I hear or read those words, I think of her. These past days, weeks, and months have been no exception. If anyone should get a pass from doing good right now, it should be Laurie. In fact, I don't care if she does well, I just want her to *be* well. I don't care if she does good, I want her to *feel* good. I sometimes find myself selfishly caring only about her world and not the big world. Because when her world is okay, this big ol' world sure seems a lot better too.

Fortunately, Laurie does not see the world so narrowly. She knows that for her world to be okay, she needs to make sure everyone else's world is okay too. Actually, she doesn't shoot for just okay; she shoots for even better. And unlike me, she succeeds. Since I met her moons ago, she's made my life even better. She makes me want to not just do good, but do better every single day. Not surprisingly, my better days of doing good have increased tenfold since I became Laurie's sidekick.

This "doing good" business with Laurie is as much a part of her as the color of her eyes and the sound of her laugh. It's innate and can't be stopped, despite all my attempts to do so. But doing well and doing good allow Laurie to transcend the challenges, the difficulties, the valleys. When she focuses on doing good, then her world doesn't get defined by the hurdle in front of her. Even when every bone in her body aches, her head feels like it's splitting open, and her mouth burns with blisters, she finds a way to do something good for somebody. Even when her new pals F, E, and C run through her body beating her up, and hopefully pummeling every cancer cell within her, she can get up and bring sunshine to someone else. She smiles, and everyone smiles with her. She laughs, and every single person can't help but join in. She does good, and when she does so, we all do better.

The Bible tells us in Galatians 6:9, "Let us not become weary in doing good, for at the proper time we will reap a harvest if we do not give up." Laurie never grows weary of doing good. Never. As I've told you, our fighter doesn't give up. May she soon reap all the good that she has sown.

We're promised that there are plans for us, plans filled with hope and a future. And as I look at Laurie, playing with the pets, laughing on the phone with a friend, persevering in spite of the poison, I know that she will reap, she will have a future, and she will keep on doing good. And in doing good, we will all be better. Amen.

From the bottom of our grateful hearts, Happy New Year, dear army! Go out and do good!

House Arrest
January 11, 2013

So our girl has finally turned a corner on the side effects of FEC. She actually began to turn this past Saturday and has really hit her stride this week. As always, she amazes me with her superhuman strength and ability to reach deep and jump the next hurdle in front of her. This time, one of the hurdles was me: I put her under house arrest, and as you can well imagine, that went over like a brick. Laurie Roth is not to be tied down—ever.

Laurie's Journey

For four or five days she felt so miserable that she didn't feel like going anywhere anyway, so I could put off telling her she was confined to our premises. I was dreading uttering the actual words, knowing the resistance our champ would put forth. After all, Laurie has specific goals of how she will get through the times in the valleys: she will continue to live life as normally as possible. She will walk the dogs, she will meet up with friends, she will pretty much do what she wants, when she wants. So you can see why telling Miss Busy Pants that she was confined to our house was the last thing I wanted to do. I considered mailing it to her in a Hallmark card. Rest assured, I will always take the chicken's way out!

I then got some help when we went to the doctor and found out that Laurie's white blood cells were basically nonexistent. Even Dr. M. went out on a limb and told her that she was going to have to "lay low." I whispered to him, "You're going to have to be a lot more specific than that, dear doctor." He acted like he didn't hear me. Even Dr. M. didn't want to try to confine our tiger. Smart man.

When we got into the car, I gently said, "You know what 'lay low' means, right?" I immediately wondered why I hadn't said this while we were still in the cancer center, where I would have had witnesses. Just then Laurie replied that she knew what "lay low" meant, but she'd "play it by ear." And that, dear army, was the sound of a line drive being hit right at the pitcher! "Play it by ear" usually means "not a chance." Oh, boy. We were now playing hardball. In all our fourteen years, not one day or minute had been spent playing fast-pitch hardball. This was probably not going to end well. None of our sports challenges ever have.

But while our champ is a toughie, she is also the most reasonable person ever made. She knew that it was best that she stay out of stores, stay away from people, stay home. While confining Laurie to the four walls of our home is akin to herding cats, she allowed it to happen for almost a week. Without white blood cells, she was vulnerable to any little germ, and she knew it. Laurie may not have wanted to stay home, but more important, she sure didn't want to end up in the hospital. So she followed my wishes: she didn't answer the door if the doorbell rang, antibacterial wipes became her BFFs, and she turned down invitations from many of you who hoped to see our girl and give her a hug.

And that was the hardest part for Laurie. She knows that without her army, this battle would be even more of an uphill climb. She knows she needs every single soldier, and each of you has never once failed to deliver. You stand by our side, you stand from afar, you always, always stand in spirit with us. You are more appreciated than words could ever tell you. Because of how important you are, Laurie lives to see you, hear from you, be with you. But I knew you would understand. I kept reminding her: "Your army understands that you can't see them right now. They understand that you are so susceptible to germs. They understand that your sidekick has channeled General MacArthur, and nobody is going to get close to you!" So if you were one of the ones that Laurie so reluctantly turned down, blame me.

The good news is that we made it through that very vulnerable time. We made it without Laurie getting sick, and that is a victory of the biggest kind. In the midst of flu bugs flying around, with negligible white blood cells and a sidekick who works in an office that's as germy as a petri dish, Laurie Roth stayed healthy! Yee-hah, y'all! (Wow, how I've missed my inner cowpoke! Haven't you? Don't answer that.)

It wasn't all fun and games, though. Her mouth sores were awful—worse than I have ever seen. If you think about that for even a second, that speaks volumes as to what they were like. They covered her tongue; they appeared all over her mouth; they were blisters of the worst kind. But eight days into it, they finally left. The pain in her bones and joints was terrible. She winced when she sat down, when she got up, even when she moved in her sleep. Yet every day, she walked Journey and Harbour down the trail, around the neighborhood, or at the park. Their life is to stay normal and when it is, so is ours.

We'll have "normal" for another week or so. Laurie goes back to the chemo room next Thursday, January 17. She will go and take the poison, knowing full well what is coming down the pike for her. As I've often said, chemo side effects become very predictable, and now we know which ones will be arriving on day three after chemo, on day five, and on day seven. But we also know that after they will arrive, they will mess with our girl, she will fight, and they will leave. The hope and prayer is that the cancer cells are also leaving. Please make that your hope and prayer too.

Thank you for your love and support. Your cards make our mailman's bag so very heavy and our hearts so very light. You carry us when we are weary. You celebrate when we are strong. You're not called Laurie's Lifesavers by accident! You are the best, and we thank our God for you every single day.

Angels Beside Us
January 17, 2013

Today was round two of our champ's date with FEC. The triple threat is racing through her and demolishing everything in the way—even the good things. We know now how these drugs work. They'll knock down her white blood cells, they'll rock her platelets, and they'll do quite a number on all the other good cells. FEC is kind of a bull in a china shop, or me on Rollerblades—pretty much everyone anywhere close to me is in danger. Same goes for FEC. The good news is that FEC approaches the bad cells with that same sense of wild abandon. No matter where those cancer cells are, FEC is on a search-and-destroy mission to find them. Those good guys will look for all the bad guys hiding in any nook and cranny of Laurie. As the nurse administered the first bags, I prayed a silent prayer as a hint to FEC to head straight for Laurie's liver and knock the crap out of those pesky cells hanging out in there. They've been freeloading long enough, and it is time to end their squatter's rights!

And as Laurie always does, today our champ found angels around us. There was a man and his wife sitting two chairs from us. She's been battling cancer for two years. Almost every week in those two years, they have spent some time at the cancer center for either her radiation, her chemo, or her appointments. He wouldn't be anywhere else but next to her. He told us their story, a love story for the ages. They met when she took a job in his insurance agency. He fell head over heels for her and worked hard to get her to feel the same way. It sounds like it didn't take long for her to figure out that this was the man of her dreams, willing to take her as his wife and her two teenagers as his very own. The fact that he was twenty-four years older than her didn't mean a thing. It was his kind smile and loving ways that she fell in love with then and that make her fall in love all over again now. We saw that smile and those loving ways all afternoon as he helped her up, as he held her hand, as he made sure those nurses watched her like a hawk. After all, this was "his girl," and she deserved nothing less.

Laurie's Journey

We sat next to Bob, who for two years has been battling melanoma, and battling it fiercely. On Christmas Eve, melanoma seemed to be winning. He was in so much pain that an ambulance had to take him to the hospital. He couldn't walk, he couldn't eat, he couldn't do anything but wonder how he would ever get through this. Six days later he went home, not in pain, one chemo under his belt and ready to fight the beast. And today here he sat, taking a second round of chemo, laughing with us, and showing pictures of the beautiful new home he and his partner, Rob, are building. I knew the second I saw the pictures of the new house under construction that my time in the conversation was going to be very short. Sure enough, within minutes he and Laurie were talking colors, trim choices, and decorating talk until my eyes glazed over. I finally backed my chair up so that it was easier for Laurie and her new BFF Bob to talk and pick out brick for the fireplace.

Since I had been edged out of Bob and Laurie's conversation, it gave me time to look at the angel beside me, the one I arrived with. It gave me time to thank our good Lord for allowing me the privilege of being her sidekick. I've been sitting next to angels all my life—first my mom, and now Laurie. I'm not sure how I got so lucky, but I assure you, every single day I say a prayer of thanks, probably a hundred times a day. It's an honor to sit beside someone so brave and courageous—to be here with her at the very place she dreads being, where she sits down, takes the bitter poison, and does so in the most beautiful way. She does it so beautifully that others are drawn to her and can't get enough of her. She bolsters their spirits, she laughs at their jokes, and she inquires so gently about how they are feeling. Even if they didn't want to talk about it, they know they'd be fools to pass up this safe haven, this angel with the kind eyes and knowing smile and soft voice who always, always asks, "How are you doing today?" They take one look at her and pour their hearts out. They tell their love stories, they talk colors, and before you know it, their chemo is done and they are on their way. My guess is that they, too, know they've been sitting by an angel.

That's how it works for our angel. She cares so much about others that she forgets she's sitting there taking her own poison, fighting her own devil, beating down her own beast. That's Laurie Roth in a nutshell. Others first, Laurie last. She's made a living out of caring for children with special needs. The kids that she has taught over the years would follow her like their own personal Pied Piper. I don't blame them a bit. After all, she's made a life out of caring for all of us, and we'd follow her anywhere, even right to the cancer center. Actually, *especially* to the cancer center. If our hero is going to be brave enough to walk into the chemo room, tuck her angel wings behind her, and take a seat, I'm going to be brave enough to watch and pray and hope to heaven above that the chemo is knocking the lights out of cancer. After all, this world needs this angel beside us every single day. It's a good world with Laurie in it. That's my world, the one I'm privileged to have, the one that I am so very thankful for every single day.

Also sitting beside us are all of you angels. You're there in spirit. (One of you named Mary even came to the cancer center and delivered a Steak 'n Shake milkshake! YUM!) You send your texts as we're walking in and sitting down. Your emails and cards arrive the week before, the week of, and the week after chemo. You are with us all the way. Our lives are lighter because your angel wings carry us through the heavy times. Thank you. Thank you so much for all your love, all your support, all the ways you show that we are not alone on this journey.

Free and Easy Chemo . . . NOT!
January 21, 2013

Just wanted to report in and let you know how things are going. Please keep our champ in your hearts and prayers. It's been a rough ride already with the second round of FEC. The side effects started right out of the blocks—no downtime whatsoever. We quickly found out that FEC does NOT stand for "free and easy chemo"! Nope, these guys are making Taxotere look like a vitamin.

We woke up Friday morning with all the regulars showing up bright and early for work. There were the severe joint aches to remind Laurie that FEC was weaving through every inch of her in search of the enemy. FEC was in such a footrace that it even caused the skin on her body to be painful with the slightest touch. She had a headache that she described as having a vise on either side of her head. It hurt to even keep her eyes open.

On Saturday, we were lulled into believing that maybe FEC had stopped being such a showoff—that maybe now it was not being so loud and boisterous about its work, but working its magic quietly and gently. Whew, we thought. Maybe all the doctors weren't kidding. Maybe this FEC regimen really is a little better tolerated. No, not so lucky; not so much. In fact, when Sunday rolled in and FEC had picked up full steam and was roaring through Laurie like a freight train off the rails, we were slammed back into chemo reality. Apparently, when they say "a little better tolerated" they are comparing it to, well, maybe a firing squad! Yes, they have us there. A firing squad might be a little worse—maybe. I really need to start asking more clarifying questions when the doctors make blanket statements like that!

Today we're at day four. Day four has brought nausea to the table, which makes Laurie immediately leave the table. FEC really could have skipped this side effect—I am perfectly capable all on my own of making Laurie nauseated with my signature dinner dishes. At least getting nauseated this way does save her the steps of politely feigning interest, taking miniscule bites, and secretly feeding Journey and Harbour under the table. But to top off this side effect, the antinausea medicine really doesn't work that well. To put it another way, the antinausea medicine doesn't work at all. But now the mouth sores have kicked in, so our girl really doesn't feel much like eating anyway. Poor thing!

So eating isn't fun, thinking of eating isn't fun, but let me tell you what is fun for our champ to think about: walking Journey and Harbour. Yes, even in this weather. Early into this marathon, Laurie said to me, "I have a goal of not missing one day of walking the girls." I knew in my heart that she would achieve this goal. I also knew that winter was approaching, it would be freezing, and I would be taking a lot of those walks with her. Walking Journey is the equivalent of walking a team of plow horses. So on days that are rough on Laurie, I get to walk (be dragged behind) Journey. If you see us out walking, Laurie is the stylish one with the cute cap and earmuffs, a neck warmer, and an adorable coat. I'm the one who resembles a cross between a bank robber and the Unabomber. By all rights, the police should be overrun with calls of a criminal on the loose as I walk through the neighborhood. I am covered from head to toe in multiple layers, a face mask that could just as easily be worn by Hannibal Lecter, a hoodie, and two pairs of gloves (a liner pair and then a pair made for snowmobiling). If I were to fall down, I have so many layers on that I would never get hurt and I would never, ever get up on my own. I would just be rolling around on the ground until a crane came and set me upright.

Laurie's Journey

Anyway, I digress. Our girl has not missed one single day. Not one! I'm sure you are not one bit surprised. I'm not surprised, but I am in awe. We got home today from our walk over at the park, and I said to her, "This is reason number 473 why you are my hero." And in true Laurie fashion, she shook her head and scoffed it off, just like the hero that she is. But I knew that she felt like crap. I knew that she could barely talk because of the sores on, under, and all over her tongue. I knew that day four had made day three look like easy street. She didn't feel like bundling up, helping me into my snowsuit, and walking Journey and Harbour for forty-five minutes in twelve-degree weather. She didn't feel like sitting upright in a chair, let alone walking the Golden Girls around Ewing Park. But my hero set a goal, and by gosh, she will achieve it—even if it does mean that she has to walk around with the Unabomber.

Walking the girls doesn't just meet a goal, it makes Laurie so very happy. She loves to see them run around, enjoying all the scents and smells and scouting out new trails for us to follow. They run ahead, then they stop and look back, as if to say, "Come on, guys, the next path is even better!" Sure enough, they're right and it is. We laugh at their enthusiastic approach to all things nature—the bird with the funny call that makes Journey stop on a dime and listen (I wish I could learn that call so that I could get Journey to stop on a dime and listen!), the little holes in the ground where they can plunge their noses and smell the little critters who make their homes deep inside, the twists and turns of deer paths that are fun for them to run down as fast as they can until they run back to their moms again. They make us laugh; they make us smile; they make us leave behind the nasty FEC side effects, if only for a little while. For just a little while, we are just out walking the dogs, just the four of us, just like we always do. I'll take "just a little while" any day of the week.

Laurie set a few other goals on this marathon: cancer would not define her, and cancer would lose. I sure like those goals! Cancer hasn't even come close to defining her. In fact, I don't think cancer has ever met the likes of our champ. No matter what it tries on her, she stands up, stares it down, and takes it on. Cancer is simply an irritant that she works through to live her beautiful life. I cling to the mental image of cancer losing, sitting defeated in the corner, possibly even whimpering because Laurie Roth has beaten the living daylights out of it. That same image is then followed by Laurie doing the most fantastic victory dance. And when Laurie finally does her victory dance, every single one of us wins. Amen.

We go back to the doctor for blood work on Thursday. Let's hope that the white blood cells have stuck around this time. We need those guys to keep our girl healthy in the face of all the flu and crazy bugs going around. I'll keep you posted!

Thank you for keeping us in your thoughts, your prayers, your hearts. We are safe there; we are protected; we are loved. Please know that we appreciate each and every one of you, and every single day we thank our God for putting you on our path and for staying with us through this journey.

You Can Come Out Now, White Blood Cells!
January 26, 2013

Well, as suspected, our champ has been fighting off the side effects of the FEC without the benefit of white blood cells. The thought of our poor girl fighting so hard with absolutely no help from her own body makes me want to BDAC (break down and cry). But as we all know, there will be no pity parties, there will be no feeling-sorry-for-ourselves days, there will be no "poor me" weeks—much to my chagrin.

Instead, there will be days that make me want to BDAC just because I live with the epitome of strength and grace in the face of all that is wrong in our lives. Just when I think that she can't take one more day of this, that her spirit is breaking and her body is following suit, she gets up, bundles up, and we're out walking in ten-degree weather. Right when I begin my prayer of "C'mon, God, please, please give her a break," she takes her head that's been in a vise all night, her stomach that has felt sick for days, and her mouth that is covered in blisters and sores, and she gets in the shower and greets the day. And just when I think that my superhero has hung up her cape and is about to give in, if only for a day, she stands up stronger and says, "Whew, I really didn't feel good yesterday, but I bet today will be better." And she makes me a believer that our day will be better too.

We have lived a charmed life in many ways. We work hard, we play harder, and we laugh a lot. We have families who love us, friends we can count on (that would be YOU!), and pets that turn a bad day into a perfect day with a touch of the paw, a wag of the tail, or a kiss right on the ol' smacker, just when we need it the most. Despite the monster inside her, Laurie makes us focus on all that is good in our lives.

When you focus on the good, the bad can't get over on you. Oh, it can get close; it can nudge right up next to you and whisper worries that you'd rather not think about. Yes, the bad stuff can do that. But Laurie reminds me that if you quickly replace those bad thoughts with all that is good, life actually becomes good again.

I can be a cynic by nature. I'm an optimist most of the time, but when I let myself, I'm a flat-out cynic. While there are many roles in the Bible that I would aspire to play, the fact remains that good ol' Doubting Thomas would probably be me in the film version. So when Laurie is hurting, in pain, crying in her sleep because her body is fighting so hard, doubt creeps in. Not that she can't beat this—never once do I think that. Never. I know that she can, and I know that she will. My doubt comes in wondering: How much can one person, this person, my person, possibly take? Did we choose too hard a road for this leg of the journey? Should we have let her body get stronger before tearing it down again? Should we have gone with a softer chemo (wow—there's a contradiction in terms!) just to let her have a rest from the cannons that have been blasting through her?

It is right at that very moment, just as doubt is beginning to take up residence inside this sidekick, when our superhero appears with her cape all neat and pressed and says, "Come on, let's walk over to the park with the dogs and play." And I look up, say a prayer of thanks, get my Unabomber outfit on, and off we go.

God truly gives His people strength when they need it the most. He knows the valleys get long, they get dark, and they sure get scary. It is then that he lifts us up to the mountaintops and allows us to survey all that is good in our lives, giving us this reminder that enables us to keep on keepin' on. He gives a superhero amazing grace so that even in the valleys, she is an example to us all. He builds steps of strength and perseverance and determination and knows his girl will climb up them, right out of the valley, and scale the mountaintop. This week, after all she's been through, as low as life was, she scaled that mountaintop, stabbed her flag into the ground, and claimed victory once again. Without an ounce of white blood cells, she fought back, fought hard, and guess what? She's winning!

We're not out of the woods yet. Her white blood cells are still very, very, dangerously low, and we have to be very, very careful. But the color is back in her face, her smile is brightening every corner of our home, and her laugh is still the best sound that I have ever heard. By maybe Monday or Tuesday, her white blood cells should start showing up like the late dinner guests that they are, and then our champ will be unstoppable. They'll slowly climb in numbers and at least help Laurie fight off the many germs that are abounding right now. We can't take too many risks, but I will get to be more of a trusty sidekick and less of a prison warden once I think she has gotten some weapons back.

Thanks for being some of our best weapons. You keep our spirits lifted, our hearts lighter, our smiles broader. Your cards, your emails, your messages and texts all help lighten the load. What an army we have assembled! Every single day we thank our Lord for each of you.

Gratitude
February 4, 2013

Hi, lifesavers—it's actually me, Laurie, at the keyboard. Do you believe it? Linda has such a way of sharing our journey with you that I tend to leave that part of it to her. But I wanted to let you know personally how much each of you means to me and what a difference you have made in my life and in this fight. My heart is full of gratitude that I will never be able to repay. I cannot get over your messages, your cards, your emails, and your prayers. I savor each one of them and read them over and over. They are truly the best medicine I could receive.

As Linda has told you, it's been a long journey with lots of challenges. I try to be very strong, but sometimes I feel very weak as the treatment wears on. There are times when I truly do wonder if I can sit down in the chemo chair another time and deal with all that comes along. I readily admit that I am not a very patient patient! Feeling poorly or unable to do some of the things I love to do does not go over very well with me. I thrive on activity and keeping busy. That's not always possible with chemo. Those are the days that make me wonder how I'll ever go back for more.

But then I get one of your wonderful cards or emails or read your posts or feel your prayers. I realize then that with your love and support, I really can do this. I not only live with a great sidekick, two wonderful golden nurses, and two funny cats (one more than the other!), but I have all of you in my corner. How lucky am I! I am reminded of why I do sit down in that chemo chair again—to enjoy all of this wonderful life that I have been given. I may have to fight for it, but when we win it, it will be oh so worth it!

So when I go sit down on February 11 for my third treatment of FEC, I bring each of you with me in spirit. You really do carry me in (with Linda pushing from behind!), and when the days get long, you carry me then too. Thank you so much. I love you all.

Laurie

Queen of Hearts
February 11, 2013

It's the ol' trusty sidekick back at the keyboard tonight. Laurie did a great job in the last update, though, didn't she? Nobody tells her story better than she does.

Speaking of telling her story, this update has to bring you up to date on what happened to our champ this past week. As some of

Laurie's Journey

you may know, when Laurie was in college, she played basketball for Illinois State University. Her time in the Redbird uniform makes up some of her best memories. Basketball helped her learn life lessons, built friendships with teammates that are still strong and intact today, and taught her that the road to victory often comes with bumps and bruises.

Recently, we had the opportunity to meet and talk to the head coach of the women's basketball team at ISU, Stephanie Glance. During that chat, some of Laurie's most recent journey was shared with Coach Glance. Breast cancer is something that Coach Glance knows all too much about, unfortunately. She was the assistant coach under the legendary North Carolina State coach, Kay Yow. Coach Yow battled cancer not once, not twice, but three times. Three times was not to be the charm, and on January 24, 2009, Coach Yow left this world and began her eternal life in heaven. The sports world and all those in her world have never, ever been the same. As legendary as Coach Yow was to women's basketball, she is also the face of breast cancer in the sports world and beyond. Her cancer fund has raised over eight million dollars, with a strong focus on research. Amen.

Coach Glance listened to Laurie's story, and I could tell she was moved by our superhero. When you hear Laurie's story told in her voice and with her words, tears stream down your face. You realize that this beautiful, graceful person is teaching us all how to do this thing called life—with a dragon breathing at her door. It was wonderful enough just to talk to Coach Glance, know that she understands the road that we are on, and see her give her sweet encouraging words and loving hug to Laurie as we parted. But Coach Glance took it another step and called Laurie early last week, asking if she would come and talk to the team at their team dinner. She also was generous enough to invite me! (That really spared everyone the nuisance of me pressing my face against all the doors of Redbird Arena, begging to be let in.)

So last Wednesday night, Laurie told her story, shared her journey, and moved us all to tears. I know her story backwards and forwards, and yet tears streamed down my face. Her gentleness is disarming when she's describing the fight of her life. Her grace is amazing as she walks you down this dark path that is lit with her smile and her laugh. Her spirit is magnetic as she reminds people, in her own unassuming way, that it's not what happens to you that matters, it's how you respond and how you recover. The ISU basketball team found out what we have all known: this beautiful being is an inspiration to us all. More than just a few of the young women on the team came up to Laurie, thanked her, and told her that they would be playing for her on Sunday. She broadened our circle that night, as only Laurie Roth can do.

Each year "Play 4Kay" games are held on basketball courts at college campuses all over the country. The players are dressed in pink uniforms and pink shoes, the coaches wear pink, and the refs often have pink whistles. Fans are encouraged to wear pink too. Proceeds of the game and many other sales go to the Kay Yow Cancer Fund. At halftime, cancer survivors are asked to come out on the court so that the crowds can recognize them, cheer for them, and be inspired by them. The ISU Redbird women's Play 4Kay game was played this past Sunday. This was the game that the girls told Laurie they would play for her. Bless their hearts.

As season ticket holders, we make most of the home games. It's been tough to do this year, with Laurie's white blood cells playing hide-and-seek. It's made this prison warden even more vigilant about limiting Laurie's contact with the outside world. But we've had a few prison breaks, and when we do, it's usually because Laurie's beloved Lady Redbirds are playing their hearts out over at Redbird Arena. Our friend Leanna is an assistant athletic director at ISU. She has spoiled us and allowed us to sit courtside for a few games. This helps me put my prison warden uniform away, knowing that we're not in the midst of all that is germy. And it allows us to escape, if only for a little while. Even a little while off this road is just what is often needed.

Well, Leanna took it up a notch for Sunday's game. She asked Laurie to help with a pregame event of presenting the game ball. This was to be done just a few minutes before tip-off, down at center court. Leanna instructed us to be behind the scorer's table when five minutes were left on the pregame clock. We are rule followers, so we dutifully went to where Leanna told us to be, excited beyond words! It's important to note that I was not going out on the court. But I am now a world famous rider of the coattails of Laurie Roth, so down I walked and took my place behind the scorer's table. I took a camera with me and acted like that's why I was there. The Redbird nation is made up of wonderful people, none of which kicked me to the curb.

Anyway, we thought that Laurie, along with Coach Glance, would present the ball *to* someone, and we were over the moon with just that prospect. With two minutes left on the clock, Laurie and Coach Glance walked out to center court—arm in arm. They were two friends bonded by two stories, sharing a day that recognizes cancer survivors and honors those who no longer are here to fight. That alone would have been emotional enough. And just as I realized that there was nobody there to present the ball to, just as I was hearing the announcer read Laurie's biography, just as the crowd was roaring and standing on their feet, I realized that Coach Glance was presenting the game ball to *Laurie*! It took

Laurie a minute for her to realize it too! But when it registered, a bigger and better smile has never been on her face!

From pretty much the minute I met Laurie, I thought that she should enter most rooms to a round of applause. I have tried to train the dogs to applaud her, but their wrists don't work that way. We substitute tail thumping (theirs, not mine), which is a great sound too. In fact, until Sunday, there was hardly a better sound that Laurie could ever have heard. But the sound of over three thousand people clapping, cheering, crying for Laurie will be a sound that neither one of us will soon forget.

On Sunday, Laurie became the queen of their hearts, like she has been to all of us. Over three thousand people saw our beautiful superhero, felt her grace and strength, and were drawn to her wonderful spirit. It was a special day for the most special of people. I will long remember Laurie's beaming smile lighting up Redbird Arena. And as icing on the cake, the Birds won!

And then came today—the third round of FEC. After ten really tough days, Laurie had actually had about ten good ones. And when you add yesterday in, she had one ridiculously awesome one! How do you go from the high of yesterday, from feeling good on the other days, from making it through the really rotten ones, to today? After all, today starts the evil calendar all over again. Day one will bring the mind-throbbing headache. On day two, Laurie's skin will feel like she has a bruise all over her body. Day three will ring in with mouth sores and blisters times a hundred. And then it tends to just get worse from there. Until finally, when day eleven arrives and you ease out of bed, you realize that the storm has passed and it's safe to peek out the windows. At least one of the monsters, the one that is allegedly on your team, has done its work and has left the building.

How do you do it? I don't know. I was the one crying today. I was the one whose heart was pounding and actually hurting at the prospect of Laurie having to sit down again in that darn chemo chair. I was the one who was choking back the words "Let's do anything but this!"

But I do know how Laurie does it. While she did shed some tears this morning, absolutely dreading what was coming, she knew she had to go. But the prospect of getting sick all over again was not in her game plan. Laurie's life isn't supposed to have this speed bump in it. She is "green for go" 24/7, and this chemo stuff is really getting in the way. So she cries for a minute, bucks up, bucks her sidekick up, and out we go. She stands tall, she walks in, and she takes the poison. She smiles and laughs and makes the nurses' and the other patients' day go so fast and so fun. She walks out and we get in the car, and she still manages to laugh at one of my stupid jokes. Who laughs after chemo? Laurie laughs, and when she does, I'm reminded of all things good, all things beautiful, all things that this life is about. Living.

Infinite Inspiration
February 17, 2013

It's been a week much like we predicted—mouth sores, blisters, skin cracks, and nausea. Chemo is so very predictable but oh, how familiarity breeds contempt. In fact, we are very ready for chemo's nasty side effects to turn down the party music and leave!

This particular week was a little different—a trickster week in a way. It started out slow, lulling us into believing that maybe, just maybe, we might dodge this awful bullet. That is not to say that Laurie was on easy street—no way—nobody gets off easy like that. But initially, the headaches seemed less intense, the body aches weren't as excruciating, and while her skin hurt, it didn't hurt every time it was touched or every time she moved. Yes, these are considered good days. The mouth sores moved in on Wednesday night, and while Laurie couldn't talk, they weren't as bad as we had seen. We began to feel downright sassy that this might be a good week—that maybe ol' FEC wasn't so FRD (freakin' ridiculously hard)!

Then Thursday rolled in . . . hello, third day. You remain the meanest day of all. The mouth sores couldn't be counted, and the blisters riddled Laurie's tongue, cheeks, and throat. Then as if that wasn't enough, the nausea built through Friday and part of Saturday. It was a teaser, though, because it never came to fruition. But I'm not sure what's worse—getting sick or just feeling like you could get sick every minute of the day? There is no good answer to this awful question.

Throughout the weekend, Laurie still proved why she's the one wearing the cape and I'm the one tying it around her shoulders. She got up out of bed, faced each day, and made sure that the two of us had more laughs than tears. She cleaned the house and made sure that we gave the dogs a good ol' walk, and then we came home to make delicious meals that probably only I will eat this week.

Today was the topper. She woke up slowly, and she even admitted to feeling poorly. Her giddyup was nowhere to be found. She still showered, she still made her usual awesome Sunday breakfast, and we still had a lot of laughs, but I could tell that she was dragging. She said to me, "This is going to be a low-energy day. I'm feeling really beat." My guess was that her white blood cells were bottoming out, as is tradition. My guess was that she would feel like the train had crashed into the station, since we had seen this before.

Laurie's Journey

My guess was that I might get to watch an afternoon of basketball on the couch with my BFFs, Ruffles and Pepsi, right by my side!

Just as I had reached into the snack cabinet, just as I had muttered "Why don't we just lie low today," just as I was about to do my launch onto the couch in front of ESPN, I heard Laurie say, "I think we need to take it easy—maybe today is the day we move that furniture in the basement." Come again? Say what? I thought you said you were tired? Who moves furniture when they're tired? Clearly, I had misunderstood her.

So we moved furniture today. I'd love to tell you that we moved mainly little end tables and lamps. My back would love to tell you that it didn't involve any sofas (two) or any chairs (four). And my legs would love to tell you that it didn't include any stairs (fourteen). As I reach for the Tylenol and my heating pad, I need to tell you that it involved all of those and then some. I'm hoping that I'm walking upright by morning.

How's Laurie doing, you ask? Fit as a fiddle! I have never seen anything like it in my life! The one with chemo ripping through her veins, the one feeling like crud long before we started, the one who doesn't have a white blood cell anywhere in her body, is doing great! I live with Superwoman and the Energizer Bunny all rolled into one. She is infinitely inspirational. If my legs didn't ache and my back worked and my hands weren't sore, I'd give her the standing ovation I believe she deserves every time she enters a room. Instead, I tell her that I owe her a round of applause, and I'll make good on it as soon as I'm off the Extra Strength Tylenol!

We pray that this week goes better. May it be a week when she doesn't have to force herself to smile, to eat, to move furniture just to show cancer who is in charge. After all, Laurie Roth deserves to live this beautiful life that she has been given. When she does, we all put a new notch in the victory column!

We will keep you posted on how things go with this treatment. Your prayers and your love are two more parts of our lives that are infinitely inspirational. Thank you so very much!

White Blood Cells Make All the Difference!
February 23, 2013

It's been a long week for our girl, and it had nothing to do with the fact that we moved three rooms of furniture on Sunday. Yes, I'm still on that. Actually, that little four-hour exercise impacted me much more than it did her! I'm still dosing up on Tylenol and complaining to anyone who will listen (feel free to ignore my incessant calls—I can easily complain on your voice mail). But nope, that wasn't the problem for Laurie. It had everything to do with a lack of white blood cells and a lack of platelets. Those two guys are very important to your immune system, your energy system, and your everything system. Apparently, the platelets decided that if the white blood cells were taking a break, they would too. Uh-oh.

We found out this news when we went for blood work last Monday. Our nurse read the report, grimaced, and handed Laurie two face masks. We knew that was code for "You have no white blood cells," but we made her tell us anyway. We were prepared to hear that the white blood cells had checked out, because they always do. But then she told us that the platelets weren't looking so hot either. That was a new one, a not-so-good one, a really scary one.

Laurie's Journey

But it makes perfect sense when we consider the number of chemo rounds that poor Laurie has been on. These continual doses do a number on her bone marrow, the major producer of white blood cells and the number one producer of platelets. As more and more chemo weakens Laurie's bone marrow, it takes longer for her little bone marrow friends to make new white blood cells and platelets. These poor guys have been working overtime for months. They probably feel like me after moving furniture! (I knew I could weave my woes in there another time.)

Some people don't rebound; their bone marrow guys quit midway through their shift, walk out with their lunch pails, and don't look back. It is no surprise that our girl's body is not made up of quitters—it's made up of all winners. Even her overworked little bone marrow guys won't take a break on her. They keep on plugging away, because they are in the body of a champion—and I bet they love her as much as all of us.

So while Monday, Tuesday, and Wednesday were absolutely awful for our girl, her body was working hard to help her. Her bone marrow guys were plugging along, working hard, pushing through the day and night to bring her counts up. Sure enough, their overtime paid off. Just when I thought that turning the corner wasn't going to happen this time; just when I wondered how long my hero could go with no energy, a lot of bone aches, and far too many mouth sores; just when I worried that we might have to go back to the cancer center and suggest a hydration or a blood infusion (a frightening thought, given how vulnerable she is to any little germ anywhere)—just then, right then, the bone marrow boys sounded the whistle that their work was done. The crew leader whispered in Laurie's sleeping ear, "Hey, Champ, we got your back!" More important, they got *her* back!

And back she came. Along came Thursday, and from the second she woke up, she seemed so much better. Not 100 percent, maybe not even 75 percent, but what Laurie Roth can do with even 50 percent is akin to a five-man construction crew. Her color looked better, the mouth sores and tongue sores were better, and the hundred deep paper cut–like sores that, for whatever evil reason, form on her fingers and hands were healing. I saw that glimmer in her eye that means one thing and one thing only: "I'm going to paint the bathroom!" Thank you, bone marrow boys—you're getting a big ol' bonus in your next paycheck!

You won't be one bit surprised to hear that with the lowest of energy, the Golden Girls still got walked every single day. Laurie's record of most consistent dog walker in the universe is still very much intact. These four-legged RNs are doing their part at keeping Laurie moving, smiling, and very often laughing. Harbour's healing energy is amazing as she walks right by Laurie's side, lovingly looking up at her with brown, soulful eyes that say, "I'm right here, Mom. You can lean on me." I really think that if it wouldn't confuse her, we should change Harbour's name to Mother Teresa. She is that kind, that sweet, that loving. Actually, now that I think about it, we could name her Laurie. Talk about confusing!

Journey, on the other hand, is sheer energy, exuberance, and enthusiasm—all healing in her own special way. She makes Laurie laugh, mainly because I am on the other end of the leash. Why is this funny? Oh, maybe because Journey pulls me, yanks my shoulder out of place, and whips me around like a rag doll as we walk through the neighborhood, down the trail, and at the park. Is it any wonder that I prefer to walk in the cover of darkness? I don't remember Journey ever doing that when Laurie held her leash. And I have to admit, it does add a lot of credence to Laurie's theory that I am the Omega to all of the Alpha pets in this house, including Sir Hobo, the resident rodeo clown!

But walking Journey the easiest thing I can do if it gives me the sound of Laurie's laugh. If I can crack her up, then it is all worth it. In this house, laughter is one of our best medicines, and we want to keep upping the dosage.

Don't let me fool you, though—Laurie is still vulnerable, still puny sometimes, and still not feeling at the top of her game. Fatigue has never been her friend, and yet that's the one hanging around the most. Isn't that always the way? The one that you could kind of do with a little less of is the one that can't get enough of you? But we're light-years from where we were even just on Tuesday, and for that we are grateful, for that we are appreciative, for that we are thankful. God delivered the energy when it was right—His timing is perfect.

And your timing is perfect—your cards, your texts, your emails all add up to bolstering our weary spirits right when we need them lifted. You are our lifesavers, you are our army, you are God's greatest gifts in our lives. Thank you.

Let's hear it for the bone marrow boys, let's hear it for you, let's hear it for our champ who keeps on swinging, fighting, living! AMEN!

On the Road Again
March 3, 2013

We wanted to check in and ask for specific prayers and positive energy points. We return to Houston on Tuesday, get scanned and tested on Wednesday, and get the results on Thursday. Hello, scanxiety!

We work very hard to stay focused on all of the blessings in our lives. We remain thankful for how God hardwired Laurie—with such strength, such fortitude, such grace. I know that I am biased, but never have I seen someone face down a beast like Laurie Roth does every day. There has not been one day when cancer has been allowed to put a notch in its victory column. Not one. Every single day declares Laurie the winner and cancer the loser. With sheer determination, Laurie proves day in and day out that it picked the wrong person. Not only did it pick my person (a big no-no), but it picked the one who has been doing life right since she landed here. If unconditional love, kindness, and a gentle spirit could beat cancer, then Laurie would have had this wrapped up in an hour. Unfortunately, we know it takes bigger weapons. Bigger weapons, meaner weapons, scarier weapons.

These weapons that we need take our champ down to depths that are so hard to recover from. There are no words to adequately convey how low chemo makes you go. It's painful; it scares you; it weakens you. As only an observer, I have been on the constant verge of crying "uncle," slapping the mat, and begging for mercy, and I'm not the one with chemo going through me. But not Laurie. Oh, I'm sure if she had her druthers, she would ride out of Dodge and never look back. But this quiet spirit doesn't know the word "quit." My hero puts her cape on every single day to go out and save our world. Thank you, Lord!

But if I told you that we remain focused on nothing but good vibes and positive thoughts as we approach next week, I would be lying through my teeth. We try to put our trust in God, and we know that He will carry us. But it's me, and God knows that I slink and sink into the "uh-ohs" routinely. Most people have "aha" moments; I have "uh-oh" moments. Examples: Uh-oh, Laurie's going to know that I ate all of the potato chips that we bought just two hours ago. Uh-oh, I think I just ran that red light—on purpose. Uh-oh, I think God forgot that my person needs to be healed completely.

So edging up to scanxiety week, I tripled up on my "uh-ohs." My faith seems even tinier than a mustard seed more often than I care to admit, and these past few days have been no exception. I just can't help but remind God that we can't afford a fumble right here. We are fourth and goal, and our champ deserves a touchdown.

Laurie has done all the heavy lifting, fighting the fight with more moxie than anyone else I know and doing so with the spirit of a lamb and the heart of a lion. Even in this marathon fight of her life, she sees the good in others, believes that so many others have it so much worse, and brings amazing grace to the table every single day. If anyone deserves good news, it's our girl. But we don't always get what we deserve. And if you're like me, when you hear that, you think, "Thank goodness I'm not getting what I deserve." But Laurie deserves the best that life has to offer. She has earned the "happily ever after." She owns the eternal rights to the Lifetime Movie Network perfect ending. She deserves it all.

Hence I start my incessant begging to God: "Come on, God, give her this miracle. Give her good news. Give her a break. Do you see her, God? Do you see her putting on a front, smiling her way through the pain, making her weary arms put the dukes up for the thousandth time? It's getting old," I tell him. "She's tired, and I don't know how much more she can take," I remind him. "She needs to hang the gloves up for a while and take a breather," I repeat again and again. I'm like a heckler in the stands outside the pearly gates. I'm sure God wishes that he had either a mute button or better security.

But I'm not done. I give him my list of how we'd like this to go. I tell him that in the best of worlds, we would hear that there is no evidence of disease anywhere in her body. There are times when we are too scared to even dare dream that, and when we do, we do so with cautious optimism. I then say that the middle ground would be that FEC beat the C-R-A-P out of cancer, but we still need a few more good punches. Okay, we could work with that. Finally, the lowest rung of the ladder would be that this regimen didn't do what we hoped, and we start from ground zero with a whole new chemo. I then make a face that gives a clear signal: Trusty Sidekick Not Happy.

And just as I'm about to remind the Big Guy of all the other things that he already knows, I feel that bony hand of my angel mother squeezing my shoulder. Clearly, heaven is not too far for the long arm of Bert Jones. In her beautiful Canadian accent, she reminds me that God loved Laurie long before she rounded out our family with her beautiful spirit. He has a plan and a future, and she will get both. Yep, you got me there, Bertie. She reminds me that Laurie's shining example of how she lives her life draws people like a magnet, and this world needs her here. Her kindness, her acceptance of others, her patience (especially with me!), and her loving nature even as she fights the beast within her—all of these are what God is showcasing. Good point, Mom. She tells me that even what I consider to be our worst option is still an option, and for that, I need to be very thankful. Right again, Mum. Options are always good.

And as she always did, my mom wraps it up with her best one. She reminds me that I'm looking so far forward that I'm losing sight of the beauty of today: this day that has Laurie up and at 'em, ready to greet the day. This day that has Journey and Harbour buckled into their leashes, ready and anxious for their daily hour-long walk in the snow. This day that has Laurie laughing, Laurie smiling, Laurie living. Dang, that little Canadian did it again. You're good, Mom.

So we'll take today as it comes, and we'll give tomorrow a whirl with whatever it brings. We'll take this marathon on as we always have, one step at a time. We'll face each day, always acutely aware that we have more blessings in our lives than worries. And when we count our blessings, your names are always at the top of the list. What an army has been assembled, filled with lifelines and lifesavers! Thank you for all you do that makes such a difference in our lives.

As soon as we can, we will update you with the news that we receive. But no matter what, together, with all of you beside us, we can face anything. Buckle up, Texas—the champ and her sidekick are coming back! Yee-hah!

Houston, We Have a Problem
March 5, 2013

I'd love to tell you that I am writing to you from sunny Texas, where we anxiously await the tests and results of the upcoming week. Instead, I get to tell you that I am writing from our own home, watching the snow pile up outside our door. Thanks to winter in the great Midwest, this snowstorm cancelled flights all over, including ours.

Try as we might to go with the flow, this threw us off a bit. It's not just the preparation that you do for any trip. It's not just the disappointment that we won't have the results until heaven knows when. It's not just the emotional energy that has been building and storing up so that we could get through this entire week. It's not just the . . . well, actually, it's all of that and then some. It comes on the heels of Laurie being completely fatigued from the chemo. It comes when we have talked ourselves through many a tough day with "At least we will know on Thursday." It comes at a time when the not knowing was deafening and the thirst and the need to know was about to be quenched.

Then just like that, it was over. Flight cancelled. Tests and scans need to be rescheduled. Our need to know will be put on the back burner again. This ol' trusty sidekick was fit to be tied, and there wasn't a darn thing I could do about it. Not one cotton-pickin' thing. As you can see, my inner cowpoke is alive and well and so ready to be released, much to Laurie's chagrin.

So we had some choices. I voted for a pity party. In fact, being from Chicago, I voted early and often for the pity party to win. Laurie, however, holds the trump card, rightfully so, and she voted that we move constructively through this bend in the road. Oh, no. I feared we were going to paint something or build something or vacuum something. Seriously, is there not another way of coping that doesn't require so much energy?

Instead, she surprised me, and this did not involve any power tools—just the phone and the computer, so that we could say what I have been dying to say to someone there: Houston, we have a problem. And they are working on the problem, working to get us new appointments, and working to see us very soon. While this is an arduous process, it has kept us moving, focused on the prize, still daring to dream of all our options.

Disappointed? Yes. Emotionally exhausted? Yep. Ready to go when MD Anderson says come? You'd better believe it. And when we go, Laurie will be that much stronger, that much healthier, and, we pray to the good Lord above, those scans will be that much better.

We will let you know as soon as we know when our next trip is scheduled. Thank you for all of your love and support. You mean the world to both of us!

There's No Place Like Home
March 6, 2013

We wanted to update you with where things are after this very long week. Wait, it's only Wednesday—it feels like it should be Wednesday of NEXT week, that's how long this week seems to have been.

After innumerable phone calls and emails, we finally got some dates from MD Anderson as to when they could scan and test Laurie. Unfortunately, their dates were about two to three weeks away. I know two or three weeks can whiz by like a rocket, and in the greater scheme of things, it really isn't that long. But when you have waited so long already, when your adrenaline has been pumped up for a while, when you absolutely need to know how the battle is going, two to three weeks seems like forever.

And there is no bullying, charming, or begging MD Anderson—heaven knows I tried all three tactics. Clearly, they have seen it all, and I am an amateur in their world. The appointment is when they say it is, and there is absolutely no wiggle room. When I told Laurie the dates that they could fit us in, the look on her face made my heart break in two. This picture of courage, this poster child for best face forward, this hero of mine who doesn't know the meaning of "quit" showed her human side. Her face fell, some tears fell, and her cape slipped off a bit from Superwoman's heavy shoulders.

Tears really haven't been part of our team. Falling faces haven't been seen too much either. And that Superwoman cape? That's usually on as tight as can be, with shoulders squared. Laurie's always ready and willing to save our world.

But even Superwoman has her moments. That moment came at about 5:00 yesterday afternoon, when we finally heard the dates and times—the dates and times that said we won't know where we stand against the beast for far too long. It was too long, and the mere look on her face told me that. The warrior was weary, the fighter was fatigued, the hero was losing heart. As far as I was concerned, that was not going to happen. Laurie's mental edge, strength, and fortitude has been a huge difference maker in this fight. We were not going to lose that edge now, just because a hospital we were working with happened to be thousands of miles away and unable to see us for weeks. It was time for the trusty sidekick to start kicking up some dust.

So at the crack of 8:30 this morning, I started my telephone campaign to our friends here at the Community Cancer Center. I explained our plight and asked about getting into one of the facilities here for testing. They didn't even make me nag or beg—although come to think of it, they do know me and have learned to avoid my nagging and begging, for everyone's sanity. They are very smart people.

But I think it was less about not wanting to hear me call them every hour on the hour and more about the fact that they adore Laurie. When they heard that she was going to have to go two to three more weeks, they couldn't bear it. When they learned that this beautiful spirit who lights up their waiting room and chemo room and every room in between would have to wait that long, they couldn't stand it. When I told them that this picture of strength was having a hard time seeing the light at the end of the tunnel this time they moved heaven and earth to make the testing happen. And when our pals at the cancer center want to move it and shake it, nobody does it better!

Within hours, we had heard from the hospital where the tests and scans will be run. Within hours, we knew that all of the scans would be this Friday. Within hours, we heard that our doctor would be getting the results on Tuesday, March 11, and our girl Sarah the Scheduler already had us written in for an 11:00 appointment. Thank you, hospital people. Thank you, Sarah. Thank you, Lord!

Don't worry—I've done the homework. Laurie's scans on these machines will be as high in quality as they come. We will have copies of her previous scans so that the radiologist who reads Friday's scans can compare them directly to the other ones. And when Laurie is recovering from all the stuff they put in her for all the tests, she'll do it right here at our house, with Journey and Harbour, her two golden nursemaids, along with Hobo the rodeo clown and Ali the taskmaster, who will make sure that I spoil Laurie rotten! She really should know by now that I'd have it no other way.

Texas has been wonderful, and we are so thankful to have the experts from MD Anderson on our team. We also have their stamp of approval for this little bump in the road, and they agreed to accept these scans for future treatments and recommendations. We're thankful for that as well, because they truly are some of the best of the best, and these brainiacs are all on our side!

But our decision to do the scans locally has brought more easy breathing, fewer tears, and a cape that now sits squarely on our girl's shoulders once again. One of the things that you learn on this journey is that you have very little control. You quickly learn that you have to control the things that you can and mitigate the damages. This testing situation became one of those things to both control and mitigate. If we couldn't get Mohammed to the mountain, then we'd bring the mountain to Mohammed. So on Friday at 11:00 a.m., our little Miss Mohammed will go over to the hospital and climb that mountain. She'll climb it high and climb it strong, and when she's done, she'll stick her flag in, declare this part of the journey done, and come on home. After all, there's no place like home.

And there's no army of lifesavers like you! Thank you again. We have felt your prayers and the strength of your positive energy through this long week (of three days). How blessed we are to have you in our lives! We will be in touch with the results as soon as we have them on Tuesday.

The Fight Continues
March 12, 2013

Well, it's not the news it could have been, and sure not the news it should have been. The CT scan showed that Laurie's liver tumors have grown on this regimen of chemo. They haven't exploded, they haven't taken over, but they did grow. It's very much the wrong direction for cancer to move.

As you can imagine, this is discouraging news. Our hero deserves only the best. She put her dukes up, kept them up, and kept on fighting. She fought when most would cry "uncle." She fought when every fiber of her body said "stop." She fought and fought and fought. And now, to hear that the three rounds of FEC did not close the deal on the beast, well, that is very hard to take—so hard that it almost made the good news fall by the wayside.

The good news: the bone scan is clear! No metastasis is anywhere to be found in our hero. More nuggets of good news: the lungs are clear. And a few more good bits: no other organ is showing that cancer is setting up shop. So everyone else read my stern memo to get the heck out of Dodge, except the darn liver. Clearly, the liver and I are not speaking the same language. I am known for my diplomacy, but it is waning. In fact, I am going to make myself very clear in future communications to the cancer in Laurie's liver: GET OUT and STAY OUT!

How we do that is what we are working on right now. We have a call and an email in to our team at MD Anderson. We are anxious to hear their thoughts and ideas. In addition, we have learned of an expert in Laurie's exact type of breast cancer: Dr. Kathy. She is with Indiana University in Indianapolis and is a leader in triple negative breast cancer. She is currently leading major clinical trials, and we are looking to contact her for her insight and possible involvement.

Finally, our good ol' Dr. M., right here, has a number of tricks up his sleeve to fight this beast. He is smart enough to have us get some of the other experts to weigh in first, and then we'll go from there. Having him on our team continues to be heaven sent! We need his optimism, of which he has much for Laurie. We need his warmth and willingness to spend an hour and a half with us and go over every detail and every option. We need his confidence that Laurie will win this. Gosh, how we needed Dr. M. He made sure that we left our appointment knowing that all the doors had not slammed shut.

My sister reminded me yesterday of something that our mom always used to tell us: when one door closes, another one opens. She would remind us that when we're looking so longingly at that one door, the one that we were absolutely convinced was the right one, we may miss out on the other ones opening wide and holding even better promise. We stare at the one door that slams shut and never lift up our heads to see the other doors that have sprung open. She gave birth to three children who were experts at putting all their eggs in one basket, convinced that there was one and only one door, only one basket. The poor thing had to pull this speech out more often than I'm sure she cared to.

And today would be no exception. Mum is probably getting her bony finger ready to poke me. She knows that I stared down the door that was supposed to say "no evidence of disease anywhere." I'd have even chosen the door that said "no progression of what we saw before." But I sure didn't want the door to open that said "the liver tumors grew." Nope, that was really the door I wanted nailed shut.

Like Pandora's box or Fibber McGee's closet, this door can't be closed now that it's open. But we can't lose sight of the other doors. We must lift up our heads and look at the other ones opening up. The one in Texas, the one in Indy, the one right here, two blocks from our house. We can be thankful that there are other doors swinging wide—not everyone hears that. We can be thankful that as dark as this day is, the open doors bring great light—not everyone gets that. We can be thankful that we have a hero who doesn't know how to quit—we have always had that. Open doors equal options for our hero, which equal hope for all. Amen.

So that's the hit we took today. Our girl is disappointed, upset, and pretty shell-shocked. How could she not be? But I know my hero. Tomorrow or the next day, the pink boxing gloves will go back on, I'll tie that beautiful cape up close to her beautiful face, and she'll climb back into whatever ring she needs to go into. We just have to get through the right door to the right ring for the right chemo partner to knock this liver cancer to oblivion. Please pray specifically that we get that answer.

Well, Look What Happens to Be Behind Door Number Two
March 14, 2013

Once again, my mom was right (not that I ever doubted her). When one door shuts, another one really does open. And we didn't even have to say the magic phrase "Open Sesame." No, sir. It just swung open with a beautiful invitation for us to walk on through. I still get chills when I think about how this door came to open up. Here's the recap.

On Tuesday, after our devastating and discouraging news, Laurie and I were sitting around basically staring at each other in complete disbelief. We tried to remind each other to be thankful that we weren't chasing the beast all around her entire body. We tried to remember that although the scan wasn't perfect, it sure wasn't where we had once been when Laurie's lung, bones, and lymph nodes had lit up in October. We tried to focus on all the good that was in our lives and be so very grateful to have each of you, our wonderful pets, and this life, despite the fear running through us.

In all honesty, all the positive talk was pretty much falling on deaf ears. We needed a win in the liver tumor column, and we didn't get it. The very victory that we needed, we didn't get. SLAM! That door slammed shut, and we felt kicked to the curb.

My mom's words came back to me: stop looking at the door that YOU thought was the right one, the only one. Look around; another will open. But you have to believe, and you have to keep your head up. You won't see one darn thing hanging your head.

As I was reluctantly picking up my head, our friends Diane and Jill stopped by. They brought a beautiful flower arrangement, lots of hugs, and four very comforting, listening ears. We told them that we were waiting to hear from MD Anderson and that we were also looking into a specialist over in Indy by the name of Dr. Kathy. But we weren't sure how long it would take to get in to see her. Diane's sister, Lynne, another pal of ours, happens to be an oncology nurse in Chicago. Di said that she would run Dr. Kathy's name past Lynne, and maybe Lynne might have an in. We thanked her, but in our hearts, we thought it was a long shot.

Well, every once in a while, the long shot pays off. Wednesday was that day. Lynne not only had an in, she *got* us in! By noon on Wednesday, we had an appointment with Dr. Kathy for next Thursday, the twenty-first! Thanks to Di talking to Lynne, and Lynne getting with Dr. Kathy, the door swung open wide for us to take a little drive to Indianapolis and meet with the nationally known specialist named Dr. Kathy.

Luck? No. Chance? Nope. My good looks? Absolutely never, ever. Laurie's good looks and good deeds . . . well, we're onto something there, but I'm not sure it works that way either. If it did, we wouldn't be in this predicament, right? I think there is something bigger at work here. I am reminded of a Bible verse (Revelation 3:8) that says, "See, I have placed before you an open door that no one can shut." I kind of picture cancer trying with all its might to push the door shut and God's pinkie finger casually holding it open. Cancer is straining, it's pushing so hard. God is not even breaking a sweat—just standing there, holding the door open, letting his girl and her trusty sidekick stroll on through. Not even mean ol' cancer can shut a door where God says it is to open. Amen and AMEN!

And God not only opened door number two, he propped open door number three as well. Door number three came in a telephone consultation today with our own Dr. A. from MD Anderson. Dr. A. spoke in his calm and warm way, constantly reminding us that although this chemo did not do the trick, he has "multiple chemotherapies" in his arsenal. As he said, let's hope we don't have to use many; let's hope that we just have to use one! He recommended where we could start and gave a huge shot in the arm to both our hero and her sidekick. To hear Dr. A. say with such surety and such resolve that he has many weapons gave both Laurie and I the other shot of hope that we so desperately needed.

So we'll do our own little version of the Indy 500 to go see Dr. Kathy on Thursday. There is no doubt in my mind that this expert on Laurie's exact type of breast cancer will know the right route for us to take. Then we will weigh her recommendations with Dr. A.'s recommendations and develop the right path. Please continue to pray and visualize that we are given clarity, great direction, and the right door to walk through for the next leg of this journey.

I also ask that you please keep Laurie in your thoughts as she continues to work through the disappointment and the continued realization that this really is a marathon, not a light jog in the park. It's a marathon that she will ultimately win, of that I have absolutely no doubt. And when that beautiful face breaks the tape at the end of this awful race, we will all have notches in our victory columns. Help her hear the cheers now: come on, hero—you can do it!

Thank you for all that you are to both of us. Thank you for all of your prayers and positive thoughts. Thank you for raining down on us with your energy, your love, and your hope. You never let us drop the ball, never let us fumble, and never, ever let us quit. What a beautiful group of lifesavers you are!

Seriously?
March 19, 2013

So just when we think we have dealt with the worst of it—that we just have to get to Thursday, get to Indy, and hear from the expert—a new little wrinkle unfolds itself. And when I say "little wrinkle," that's one of my bigger understatements of 2013.

This "little wrinkle" involved Laurie being in a lot of pain for about a week. The pain was located right at the site of the larger tumor that is in her liver—just under her rib cage on the right side. That particular tumor is on the edge of the right lobe of her liver. The theory is that the growth we have seen in that particular tumor is causing it to push on the side of the liver, which then causes inflammation in the area. There is also another theory that Laurie's little white blood cell guys, who have been running for the hills on most days, are actually trying to fight off the tumor. Finally! Dr.

M. explained to us that when the white blood cell guys got in the game, they set out to do their job, which is to attack the tumor. But when they do so, they cause inflammation. Apparently these guys are making up for lost time, because there is a lot of inflammation! Thank you, little white blood cell guys. You're tardy, but clearly, "better late than never" is the phrase that comes to mind.

Anyway, the pain intensified over the weekend, and by Monday it was a fifteen on a scale of one to ten. As you would imagine, our champ has the highest pain tolerance of anyone I have ever met. She is so strong that she has always been able to muscle through anything, barely needing a Tylenol. She moves through all things painful, refraining from the theatrics that accompany my moments of even anticipated pain from, say, a stubbed toe, splinter, or paper cut. So for her to even mention that she was hurting meant that the pain was off the charts. The scarier part was that she was on some pretty strong painkillers, and they weren't touching it. Not even a little bit.

I had popped home for lunch yesterday after having a good conversation with our nurse, Katie. We were going to try a different dosage of the pain meds and hoped that would work. Laurie took the medicine, just like we had talked about. And by 3:30 the pain was worse. Seriously? This was not the direction I wanted it to go. This seemed a bit much to put on our already crowded and worried plate. This really wasn't what I had in mind for our girl. But there we were, for whatever reason, and we needed to move quickly to get things under control. So off to the emergency room we went—yes, that's how much pain Laurie was in. She actually *agreed* to go to the ER!

We arrived and, thankfully, were the only ones there, so they got us right in. We told our story to our nurse, Justin, and the ER doctor,

Dr. G. They were both wonderful. Dr. G. decided to talk to Dr. M., so we had some time with Justin. In true Laurie fashion, she got Justin to tell his story. Turns out that Justin is a cancer survivor. This six-foot-four, strapping, good-looking, gentle guy had the scare of his thirty-seven years last April, when a tumor was found that stretched from one side of his chest to the other, intertwined in his heart. That tumor was malignant, and it had to be reduced because it couldn't be surgically removed. That tumor is now gone. Justin praised his doctors, calling them the best, the best who saved his life.

And where did Justin get his treatment? Where did this nurse who works at our local hospital, who lives in a nearby small town, who is a local boy, go for his treatment? Wait for it . . . Indiana University Simon Cancer Center, where we are going on Thursday. Coincidence? No. Unbelievable? Almost. Just what we needed to hear? You better believe it! Justin told us his wonderful, miraculous story, praising the doctors at IU and giving them all the credit for why he was standing there taking care of us. And in doing so, he gave us another shot in the arm and a big dose of hope that we needed.

I began to wonder if maybe this, and this alone, was the really good reason why we had to go to the ER and get Laurie's pain under control. It was beginning to make more sense to me that what had made me so upset—for Laurie to have to expend her precious energy, sit in a germy ER (it was actually very clean, I'm just a germophobe who should have bought stock in Lysol years ago), and be anywhere but home, where I love her to be—was now unfolding a story of hope, of strength, of survivorship. Maybe? Probably? Absolutely yes. Once again, there are angels on our path every step of the way. Add Justin to that ever-growing list.

Anyway, Dr. G. came back in the room and had Dr. M. on the phone. Dr. M wanted to talk to Laurie about our options. Partway through that conversation, he told Laurie that he was almost to the hospital and would see her in a few minutes. What an angel we have in our Dr. M.! After a long day in the office, he was going to spend some free time with Laurie. And in he came, with a big smile, great laugh, and warm heart that immediately made us feel that things were soon going to be under control. Oh, how we needed some control!

He set out a couple of different options for Laurie. Option one: She could stay in the hospital and get a pain pump. It would take about twenty-four to forty-eight hours, and that would get her over the hump that the oral stuff might not be able to do on its own. Option two: We would wait to see the effects of the pain shots that Laurie was given in the ER (two big-boy shots that would have sent me to Pluto for the next three months without any audible abilities, and yet here was Laurie conversing with the staff). If the shots worked, then we could go home with two new pain meds to combine with the other one that we had been given. Option two ended up working out—Laurie's pain was reduced to a manageable level (well, if you consider an eight a manageable level), she could actually walk upright (a feat she had not been able to do when we arrived), and was able to breathe without moaning. Breathing is pretty essential, so it was important that we got that piece right.

So home she came. Home to the best golden nurses in the land (sorry, Justin, you're really good, but nobody holds a candle to Florence Nightingale's sisters, Journey and Harbour). Home to a little rodeo clown named Hobo, who makes Mama laugh, and now laughing doesn't cause too much pain. Home to Alicat, who sensed that it was no time to bite Mom and instead sat behind her on the back of her chair, keeping her eye on the prize of our household. Home. Thank you, Lord, for letting me bring the heart of our home right where we always must have her: home.

We were up during the night for a little over an hour, because Laurie felt sick to her stomach. I'm sure it has something to do with the fact that she had enough pain medication to knock down a team of plow horses. But we have to keep the meds going. This pain medication regimen will keep up until we get the pain better managed. So while she is under the influence, I'll be fielding phone calls, signing important documents, and doing all of the driving. This is no time for our own personal Janis Joplin to get involved! My hope is that she will sleep. Sleep is good. Sleep is healing. Sleep is what our superhero needs so she can continue to save our world.

So that's the news. Please continue to pray and think positive thoughts that Laurie's pain will remain managed. That we will get to Indy, get to Dr. M., and get the plan that beats the beast into oblivion. That we will continue to find beautiful angels along our path—angels like you who hold us, carry us, love us. From the bottom of our grateful hearts, thank you.

Options—What a Beautiful Word
March 21, 2013

Well, we have a few more angels to add to our ever-growing list. Let's add Dr. Kathy and Cheri, her research specialist and RN. Their kindness, comforting manner, and excellent expertise are coming onto the team at just the right time.

As I mentioned before, Laurie has a very specific type of breast cancer. Hers is called triple negative breast cancer (TNBC). How dare something so awful sounding (and acting) be taking up residence in such a beautiful person! This TNBC is a rough one, and scientists, researchers, and pharmaceutical companies are working hard to crack its code. If given a chance, I'd like to crack more than its code! But I digress.

We are thankful that the doctors at MD Anderson figured out that we are not dealing with just a run-of-the-mill breast cancer. While run-of-the-mill breast cancer is no walk in the park, there have been steady and significant strides made to make it more manageable. TNBC has eluded such a step.

Enter Dr. Kathy at IU Simon Cancer Center. She has been on the tail of TNBC for years. She has spoken at national symposiums, raised awareness, raised funds, and raised Cain about this type of breast cancer. She has been like a bounty hunter chasing down a fugitive at large— forgoing sleep, showing its picture around the nation, talking about this runaway to anyone who would listen. Boy, are they listening. TNBC is now in the forefront of many researchers' minds and a top line item in the budgets of the pharmaceutical companies. Thanks to Dr. Kathy and her dedicated group of colleagues across the nation, the fight against TNBC now has lots of viable options.

And when the fight has lots of options, so does Laurie. Amen. That's what we heard today: "You have lots of options." More beautiful words have rarely been spoken. Then, after we began breathing again after hearing those words, Dr. Kathy said, "Now, let's narrow this down and figure out where to start." Hello, angel.

Dr. Kathy gave us two separate options to consider right out of the box. There was so much to think about, so much to process, so much to work through. Rather than rush through this important decision, we decided that we would come home, think through it, and make a decision tomorrow. Dr. Kathy thought that was a great idea. While there isn't a wrong option, since both have equal potential to do good, we just need to decide which route to take. To make sure that we had all the info to make our decision, Dr. Kathy had Cheri, her research specialist, come in and walk us through all the nuts and bolts of the options. It was if these two very busy people had nothing but time for a hero and her sidekick. That's an angel for you. Since I live with one, I know this behavior very well.

Speaking of that angel, please keep our champ in your hearts and prayers, where I know both of us are tucked so very safely. Laurie continues to have pain, and while it is nothing close to what it was on Monday, it is still there. We continue to use all of our weapons against it, and whichever future chemo option she chooses, it will be designed to shrink the tumors and relieve the pressure. The problem is that no matter how quickly we decide on the option, the earliest she will start on any treatment plan is late next week. So we ask for your prayers and positive thoughts that we can manage the pain and let our girl have her good days back.

We will keep you posted on what we decide and where we will go from here. The doors keep opening, and the angels just keep walking through them bringing new options to the table. We are blessed to have the doors, the options, and all of you angels. Thank you so very much!

Racing for the Cure!
March 25, 2013

As we have said many times, this journey that we have been on since May 2012 has been more of a marathon than a light jog around the park. A marathon is well known for pushing people past the normal limits of human endurance and testing their mental fortitude to deal with all 26.2 miles of the grueling contest. It will come as no surprise that I have never, ever entertained the slightest thought of participating in a marathon. In fact, I don't even like to drive 26.2 miles, so you sure as heck are not going to see me running it.

But Laurie? There is a marathon runner built inside her. She has the strength to stay the course and the focus to avoid being distracted by an unforeseen or disappointing turn of events. She has a resilience that allows her to bounce back from pain, discouragement, and obstacles so big that they seem to be not just hurdles, but complete show stoppers. Within Laurie is the person who knows that every journey, every race, every marathon is a series of steps, some easier than others, some almost impossible, but all leading one step closer to the goal.

And that goal for Laurie is life. Laurie, thank goodness, is willing to accept no other vision. The image in front of her that keeps her taking one painful step after another is the picture of her beautiful life: the life with a trusty sidekick, two golden nursemaids named Journey and Harbour, a homegrown comedian cat named Hobo, and a "kickin' tail and taking names" cat named Ali; the life with two families (hers and mine) that adore her and truly believe that she hung the moon; the life with a host of friends who feel like family and who are really angels, made up of each of you.

Long ago, Laurie designed a life that all of us could only hope to have. Her life epitomizes the Golden Rule (canine foreshadowing, apparently), as she leaves no heart unturned and always makes sure people know how much she loves them. From the small children she taught, to the sidekick who acts far too much like those children, every single person has always known that Laurie Roth was a difference maker in their lives. She has been a gentle holder of hearts, willing you to be better, to be stronger than you know, to be the change that we need to see in this world. Throughout this journey, I have marveled at her strength, her drive, and her mental toughness in the face of the beast knocking down our door. She has adopted the words of the legendary coach Kay Yow: when life kicks you, let it kick you forward.

And being kicked has sure happened all week since I last wrote. Try as we might to get the pain in her side to go away, it's still there. The overall fatigue and just-not-feeling-great remain. Bless her heart—when I ask Laurie to rate her pain, she will honestly say, "Oh, about an eight. But that's not so bad." Not so bad? What is she comparing this to? Bamboo shoots under her fingernails? Mind you, this eight is WITH the pain medicine. I then inquire how an eight could be "not so bad," and Laurie reminds me that last Monday it was a fifteen. Okay, she's got me there. What an angel, what a fighter, what a hero.

It's been a tough week, but she kept moving, kept walking Journey and Harbour, kept smiling. She may have been kicked, but cancer wasn't going to see her sweat. She may have been kicked, but she was not down, and she sure wasn't out. She may have been kicked, but her eyes were on the prize and the only goal she knows: life.

So forward we go. Forward to Wednesday morning. This Wednesday morning, Laurie will need every angel in her army, every bit of strength within her will, and every ounce of her unflinching sense of focus to continue on this marathon. It is on Wednesday morning that we will walk back into the cancer center for Laurie to sit down and take the new chemo. This new chemo is named Cisplatin—finally, a slightly nicer-sounding chemo, if there is such a thing. It was one of the two choices that we had, and we're going with this one. It will more than likely kick her; they all seem to have that trait. Our prayer and our hope is that it kicks her forward, right across the finish line.

We plan to frequently test this one through blood work and other lab tests, as well as CT scans if things don't seem right. The new plan for this new leg of the marathon is to test early and often. Speaking of kicking, I am going to have Laurie visualize kicking the bejeebers out of cancer. It is high time that it vacates its squatter's rights and lets Laurie get back to this beautiful life she so purposefully designed.

I'll keep you posted as to how our girl does. Thank you for your prayers and positive thoughts as our race to find the cure continues. Thank you for being our army of lifesavers, always marching right alongside us. Thank you, from the bottom of two very grateful hearts, for being there every step of the way. Come on, Champ—you have some kicking to do!

Hope Floats
March 27, 2013

Well, we're finally home. After about seven hours at the cancer center, multiple bags of multiple medicines, and one big bag of Cisplatin, our girl is home. Home, where the golden Florence Nightingales can do their good work. Home, where even Ali and Hobo seem content to be calm (Hobo) and nice (Ali). Home, where Laurie always should be.

When we left home this morning, we followed our usual "off to chemo" routine. We had a group hug and prayer; Journey and

Harbour are much better at bowing their heads than are the cats. Of course, tempting the girls with a couple of treats on the floor always helps the bowing-of-the-heads trick. We had the cancer center bag all packed; since we first walked through those doors many moons ago, we have used the same bag, a pink-striped Reebok breast cancer bag that holds all our essentials. We pack at least one iPad, a book, and magazines; various pictures of the pets, family, and friends for Laurie to use for visualization and comfort as the chemo goes through; and some gum (for Laurie) and a Pepsi (for me).

Today I threw in two other items: two inspirational stones that we usually keep on the fireplace by the sunroom door, right where we can see them the most and be reminded of them. One of the rocks is etched with the Teddy Roosevelt quote, "Believe you can and you are halfway there." Amen, Teddy. This marathon is almost as much mental as it is medical. Sometimes the mental may win out before the medical. Any of our doctors or nurses would confirm this. They marvel at Laurie's mental fortitude—that fierce spirit from this gentle soul who fights on, fights well, fights through. Her mental place has given her the edge more times than anything else. And as hard as that is to sustain, now more than ever we have to keep that up. We must continue to believe that we can and let that carry us halfway, and then go all the way across that finish line.

The other rock was given to us by our dear friend Judy, and it says what we must also always sustain: HOPE. It's powerful in its simplicity. It is what we must have, must sustain, must believe. Hope. We have been promised hope and a future, and I'm going to hold God to that.

By the time I had carried the bag from the car into the cancer center, I was really regretting tossing two rocks into it. What was

Laurie's Journey

I thinking? I'm not sure if you are aware of this, but just so you don't make the same mistake I did, here's a news flash: rocks are heavy—even cute ones that are etched with great words. I made a mental note that next time, I'm just going to jot the words down and read them to Laurie. That approach might lose a little on the visualization piece, but I will save a boatload in Advil and massage therapy costs.

Anyway, in we went, Laurie trying to smile, me trying to be positive for our girl. We weren't fooling a soul—not one single soul, and certainly not each other. We were doing the very thing we never, ever wanted to do again. We were walking through the doors of the very place we never wanted to go back to. We didn't want to be there, and yet we had to be there. Today would start our new regimen. Today would start the new fight with the old beast. Today was the start of all our new hope.

You know you've been to a place far too much when you walk in and you're greeted like Norm at Cheers. As fun as that is, the place where you want everybody to know your name is not the cancer center. But our team there does. They are now old friends, all pulling for us, hugging us when they see us, hoping right alongside us. Our hope began to float just by being with these wonderful angels who work there.

And then our friend Tina walked in, just to make us laugh, smile, and know that our lifesavers are always there for us. Soon Laurie's sister Jenny came to sit with us, to make our day go faster and so much sweeter. When the Roth girls smile, it lights up the darkest of rooms. So imagine the light coming into the chemo room from Laurie's and Jenny's beautiful smiles. They could have turned off the lights and the room would have been perfectly illuminated. Around lunchtime, in walked our dear friend Julie with a bag of food and treats and love. Behind her came our sweet pal Pat, who spent time with us, warming us with her wonderful friendship and constant support. Thankfully, the cancer center didn't invoke the "one person with one patient" rule, which they usually do. I think they gave us a pass just for today, knowing how much our champ needed some members of her army sitting close by.

With each person, we were reminded that hope floats. It floats in our hearts and in our minds and in our souls. It floats in with one friend and then a sister, and then more friends. It floats in with your prayers and your love and your support. Hope floats, and when it does, it makes believers of all of us. Believe you can and you're halfway there. From that rock to God's ears. We must believe, we must trust, and we must always, always hope.

Rumor has it that this Cisplatin is not nearly as nice as its name kind of makes it sound. It may start with "Cis," but it's no sissy. In fact, apparently it's as mean as Laurie's other three chemo drugs combined. Yikes. It's a type of chemo agent that Laurie's cancer has never met. That's a good thing, because it means that the squatter in Laurie's liver is about to have a rude awakening.

But as it shows the cancer that there's a new sheriff in town, it will knock Laurie around a bit. Actually, it will probably knock her around a lot. The fatigue could be tough, the nausea might be worse, and it could bring other side effects that won't be one bit fun. We have weapons to try to counteract the effects, but for the most part, we will have to ride them out. My hope is that our champ weathers these side effects, that they arrive and leave in short order, and that our girl has more good days than not-so-good. Please make this your hope too.

I'll keep you posted as to how our hero does. Right now she has dozed off, and all of her nurses are around her. What a beautiful sight.

Thank you for being an army of lifesavers who make our souls soar, our hearts light, and our hopes float.

Headwind
April 1, 2013

The dictionary defines a headwind as "a wind blowing from directly in front, opposing forward motion." With that in mind, this past weekend was a full-blown headwind. No matter how we turned, the wind blew us back. We couldn't get ahead of it or around it. There was absolutely no forward motion happening. It had hurricane strength and took us both with it.

It was a headwind filled with fatigue like we've never seen. Cisplatin is famous for fatigue. Laurie was literally in bed for most of yesterday, weaker than a kitten, with little to no appetite. There is no explaining chemo fatigue. If I didn't see it in Laurie, I would just think people meant that they were *really* tired. My bet is that people with chemo fatigue would take *really* tired over this any day of the week. There's no going to bed, getting your rest, and then waking up feeling renewed and refreshed. Nope. That ain't happening. No amount of sleep is going to recharge these batteries. After all, they've been drained by a poison that's fighting for the cure. I just wish the cure didn't feel so much like the enemy.

Cisplatin's other well-known side effect is nausea. The fun really never stops with this drug. That's just what you want to feel when you're so tired you can hardly keep your eyes open—you want to have the constant feeling that you are going to get sick to your stomach. No. Not really. Not so much. We are trying to keep that wolf from the door with the antinausea drugs that we were given. We should have known that this was a bad one when they gave us not one prescription of antinausea drugs, but two! And these are on top of the multiple bags of antinausea drugs Laurie got with her chemo on Wednesday. Now we know exactly why.

This weekend was a rough one, no two ways about it. We know that Days 3 through 7 after chemo are the toughest, and Cisplatin was very punctual from that standpoint. If the chemo calendar is correct, these awful side effects will hopefully begin to wane around Wednesday. Frankly, that's far too long. And there's very little we can do about it. Laurie spent most of yesterday resting, because her body wouldn't allow anything else. I spent most of it turning the phone off, taping over the doorbell, and watching Laurie sleep. She was never in a deep sleep, because after I had been staring at her for five or ten minutes, she would slowly open her eyes and tell me she was okay. I'm sure she wanted to tell me to get another hobby, but she is far too polite to ever say anything close to that.

Even when she's so tired and so weak, she wants to make sure that I'm okay. I tell her over and over that I'll be okay when she's okay. She worries about so many others and is always saying that "things could be so much worse." And perhaps, while they could be, this truly is our worst time and the one that matters most to me. This is the one that I want us to move out of, away from, as far as we possibly can from.

I watch her try to fight through these side effects, longing for the life she had even just a few weeks ago. It wasn't perfect, but it was better than sleeping all day. Laurie Roth wasn't built to sleep her days away. She was built to be on the move. She was jam-packed with a ton of energy. She was perfectly designed to perfectly design our life, our very beautiful life. And so far, I've yet to see anyone do it better. Even on her worst days, she's a better person than most. I keep in constant conversation with God, with my mom, with anyone who will listen, and I tell them that our hero needs a break. Our champ has put her dukes up time and time again, and she's weary. We need our own Easter—the one that breathes new life into us and promises spring, promises hope, promises life. I'll forgive its tardiness if it comes even a few days late.

Let Easter come; let spring be here; let Laurie put her face to the sunshine and soak it all up. Take the headwind away; let the wind shift to our backs. Yes, that's my hope and my prayer for our girl today: that she not get pushed back, not one step back, but only pushed forward. May today be the day that she is able to, as Coach Yow always said, press on.

I'll keep you posted. Thank you for keeping us in your prayers and in your hearts. Those are the safest places that we can be.

Restless Rest
April 6, 2013

The strong headwind is still blowing hard at our house. It has blown so hard that it has kept our champ in bed a lot, weary from trying to withstand it, weak from trying to get around it. This sidekick has never felt more helpless in her life.

If I thought for one minute that all of this rest was actually helping her, I'd be so thankful that rest has come to sweet Laurie Roth. After all, this is the original Energizer Bunny, minus the obnoxious, incessantly clanging cymbals. Laurie is the one who never stopped, who always had that extra puff of steam to do one more thing, who kept our beautiful life moving in such a beautiful way. She has been infinite in her strength, her sturdiness, her stamina. This has been how Laurie has faced life; this has been how Laurie has faced everything.

So if her sleeping and resting meant that she was recharging, I would welcome this land of Nod that she has recently found. But this is a slumber that comes from nowhere good—from the heavy hits that she has taken repeatedly, from the ten rounds of chemo in as many months from which her body never got a break, from the disease that keeps nipping at her heels. She's exhausted from trying to stay one step ahead—so much so that we had to go to the cancer center yesterday and get two liters of hydration fluid pumped in, along with a bag of antinausea and steroids for good measure. That seems to be par for the Cisplatin course too—the need to go and sit for four and a half hours and be hydrated. I'm telling you what, this Cisplatin is making the other chemo drugs look like pantywaists.

On a day when Laurie was so weak, she had to go and get poked so that she could get hydrated. On a day when her soul was weary and the covers were consoling her, she had to go and put on the game face. On a day when my hero actually doubted she had the strength to walk all the way to the chemo room, she had to use up her energy to do so. What I wouldn't give to take the pokes, soothe her soul, carry her anywhere she wanted to go. What I wouldn't give to carry her so far away from the beast, from the pain, and right across that finish line. What I wouldn't do to take this all away from her and give her back the life she so perfectly designed for us to have. Unfortunately, all of us who love her so know all too well that this is not how it works. It is the single most helpless feeling in the world.

Laurie's Journey

I know you know exactly what I mean. You're feeling as helpless as I am. Not a day goes by that I don't hear from members of this big army wondering what they can do. I hear it in your voices, in your texts, in your emails: "Name it, I will do it." "I'm here for you night and day." "Whatever you guys need, consider it done." As I have said many times, you're not called Laurie's Lifesavers for nothing. We both know that if you could, you would take it all away. From the bottom of our hearts, we thank you for your love, your support, your unwavering willingness to be right by our side.

And as hollow as that may feel to you, THAT is helping. I'm not prone to regularly quoting Marlene Dietrich, but I have always loved her line, "It's the friends you can call up at 4 a.m. that matter." You got that right, Marlene. We have a whole army of friends like that, friends such as you. I know darn well that if we called, it would never go to voice mail. Thank you.

Please keep being there, praying for us, sending up positive energy to whatever spirit it is that you hold fast to. Our girl is in a valley right now. The weapon that we have is kicking her tail right and left. Her body is weary from the long fight. Her smile doesn't come quite so easily, but it is just as pretty anytime it flashes across that beautiful face of hers. I believe that God loves Laurie Roth like nobody's business. I believe that when we weather this storm, we will have sunshine again in our lives. And more than anything in the world, I believe in my hero. And in my book, my hero always, always wins. She absolutely has to. What's a sidekick without a hero to behold and brag about?

We return to the cancer center on Monday for blood work and more hydration. I will keep you posted on how our girl does. May she turn the corner, face the sun, and beat this beast into oblivion. Amen.

Not Getting Any Easier
April 9, 2013

Some days seem seventy-two hours long. Yesterday was one of those days. In fact, at one point it felt as if time stood still and a bad dream began—one that neither Laurie nor I can seem to awake from.

Sunday and Monday were not any kinder to Laurie than the previous seven days had been. But despite being so tired and so weak, she pushed herself to ride to the park on Sunday with me and the Golden Girls so she could watch us walk around. She pushed herself to sit up and watch some basketball games with me. She pushed herself to have dinner, to talk, to smile. All the while I was encouraging her that on Monday we would go and get her hydrated, and that might help her feel better.

I have never been more wrong. Because while we were at the cancer center and Laurie had the bag of hydrating fluids going into her, Dr. M. came into the room. The very look on his face told me that this was not going to be a good conversation. Dr. M. loves Laurie, he enjoys her, and he admires her. Dr. M. looked like a guy who was going to have to say things to a hero that he never wanted to say. Somehow he found the words to tell us that this treatment wasn't doing for Laurie what any of us hoped it would. In fact, it seemed to be doing more harm than good.

Dr. M. explained that Laurie's liver function test results were pointing to a very serious situation. They were so off the charts that it appeared we were moving into possible liver failure. We were moving into an area from which we more than likely couldn't recover. The cancer was moving at breakneck speed and yet bringing our world to a screeching halt. I seriously believe that both my heart and my world stopped for a little bit yesterday afternoon. At the very least, they both broke in two.

Dr. M. spent over two hours with us, answering every question, none to my satisfaction. He explained that while her liver wasn't consumed by the cancer, the location of the tumors was making life difficult for Laurie. Their very location was what was preventing her from taking deep breaths, or having energy, or feeling even the slightest bit better. They were pressing on things that they shouldn't have been pressing on, much like the elephant that seemed to be sitting squarely on both of our chests.

Cancer is a trickster. Many times, even when you hear that you have options and you are thankful to hear that, you realize that you have the devil in one hand and hell in the other. It was his opinion that we basically had two options: we could try another round of Cisplatin, or we could try to make life as comfortable as possible for our girl. To me, those aren't options. To me, those are our nightmare.

Cisplatin has been too much for Laurie's body. It came a bit late in the game, steamrolling over her and taking almost every ounce of her energy with it. Neither of us can fathom putting her through another round of it. And while making Laurie comfortable has always been my number one goal, this is not the way I pictured doing it. So our options are limited, our options are difficult, our options, quite frankly, are awful.

We trust Dr. M. implicitly. He has become more than just a doctor to us—he has become a friend who wears a stethoscope. But we have also been blessed to have other stethoscopes join us on our path, and I have calls in to Dr. Kathy in Indy and Dr. A. in Houston. We want their opinions of where we are at, what other options there may be, and where to turn next. We will leave no stone unturned as we race with even more urgency for the cure.

As you would guess, our hero is every bit of a hero still, despite the devastating news we heard. There have been many tears shed, many questions asked, many shakes of the head wondering how in the world our world landed here. But as only Laurie Roth can do, her inner strength, her boundless beauty, and her soft, sweet voice remain so filled with grace and courage.

Our girl deserves a better option than the ones we heard yesterday. I am praying, and I know you are too, that we hear a different option today.

Tough Days
April 15, 2013

Since I last wrote to you, we've had a lot of tough times. Times when pain has kept Laurie awake. Times that have worn her out. Times that have not led us to turning the corner like we had hoped. And then there have been other times when it seemed like Laurie's liver was trying really hard to reboot. Times when she had more strength than I could have ever imagined her showing, knowing what she was going through. Times that allowed our hope to keep floating toward us, near us, over us.

These have been quiet days at our house. Laurie is resting and sleeping to give her body every shot at fighting for her. Some of the rest comes during the day, because it has eluded her at night. Some of it comes because of the pain and the pain meds, and a body at rest is more likely to heal. So rest she does.

Laurie's Journey

We've had long talks about tough things. We've cried, and we've been afraid of where this is going. I continue to tell her that my money is on her. If anyone's body can turn this around, it is hers.

We've had walks down memory lane. Our life together is filled with so many wonderful times, more times than we can count or probably even remember. Laurie tells me over and over that she has so much to live for and that's all she wants to do. The fighter is ever present in sweet Laurie Roth. It never leaves her. It's who she is and how she's wired. Again, if anybody can turn this around, it is Laurie.

As I sit here, I don't know where this road is leading. I don't know if Laurie's poor little liver has just been so beaten up by chemo and by cancer that it is too afraid to come out of hiding. I don't know what to pray for, because I can't bear for Laurie to suffer and yet, if the corner is coming, we have to hold on. I don't know how something so evil could be growing in someone so beautiful, so good, and so kind.

What I do know is that this earth needs the smile of Laurie Roth more than heaven does. Heaven has enough of my angels, so it can leave this one here to spread the joy and love and laughter that Laurie always has spread. I do know that if anyone deserves for life to get easier for her, it's Laurie, who has always made sure that life was easier, better, and more wonderful for everyone else. I do know that if anyone deserves a miracle, it's Laurie.

I'm praying for a miracle. Please join me.

Thank you for all of your gifts and cards, your texts and emails, phone calls and messages. I let Laurie know about each of you, you beautiful members of this tireless army. You make her smile.

We appreciate and love you more than words could ever convey. Thank you so much.

Tough Days Continue
April 19, 2013

I sat down last night to update you, and the words just would not come to me. Every time I put my fingers to the keyboard, tears would stream, and I could not even begin to formulate an update to our precious lifesavers.

Part of the problem was that I was not near Laurie as I was typing. I was in another room, but I could hear her. She had her sister Jenny right by her, but for me, even a room away seemed too far. So I turned off the computer and went back to the place that has been my comfort zone for so many years: by Laurie's side.

Over the past week, things began moving very rapidly, all in the wrong direction. I connected with hospice (or as we like to call them, "supportive care," because that is what they do—they support you and care for you). They confirmed what my heart was fearing: that Laurie's liver was not coming out of hiding. It had been hit too hard far too many times, and the last hit had been lethal. The outcome that Dr. Kathy had feared was coming true: Laurie's liver was in toxic shock, and the downward spiral was moving too fast to stop.

This is how fast: On Tuesday morning, Laurie was able to talk and converse, though not for very long, and doing so took a lot out of our girl. By Wednesday afternoon, when our supportive care nurse, Linda, came to see her, words were hard to get out and staying awake was an even harder chore. I answered most of the questions, with Laurie nodding in agreement.

Yet Linda was still able to see the Laurie we all know, love, and adore. With Laurie saying barely more than five words, Linda saw her gorgeous eyes and her beautiful smile and fell immediately under the Laurie Roth spell. At the end of our meeting, as I was walking Linda out, she turned to me and said, "What an amazing and special person. I am in awe of her." Laurie's record for unassumingly stealing hearts is 100 percent intact. No surprise there.

Linda explained that in their assessment, they look at many things in the patient to determine whether these are critical times. The three biggies are circulation, blood pressure, and heart rate. The circulation is typically not very good, and Laurie's isn't. The blood pressure is usually very low, which Laurie's really isn't. And the heart rate is usually very high, which Laurie's is. In fact, Laurie's heart is doing everything it can to keep Laurie right here. Is it any wonder that of all the strength embodied in this one body, it is Laurie's heart that is still the strongest of all?

But the reality has become that these are critical times—critical times creating tough days and rough nights, days and nights that are nothing that Laurie would ever want or deem as a way of life. And that becomes the critical piece in these critical times. Laurie's life has been nothing less than top-notch quality—every aspect, every word, every deed. Despite the fear and the grief and the pain in which I face each and every minute by Laurie's side, I know that not one minute of any of the past few days would be the way Laurie would want to live. This is not Laurie's life, and I owe it to her to not be selfish (though, knowing me as she does, she would have not one single expectation for me to be the bigger person). Even though this is my nightmare, living like this would be hers.

So we are spending these days surrounded by the love of family and friends, prayers and positive thoughts, lifesavers and soldiers of this beautiful army. I am constantly reminding Laurie that she is loved, she is cared for, she is safe. All the things that she always gave to me, gave to you, gave to all of us who were lucky enough to cross her path, we can now give back to her. This beautiful, perfect person deserves nothing less.

PART 4

The Journey Continues

A Hero Is at Peace
April 20, 2013

If you noticed that a light went out of this world at 1:40 p.m. on Friday, then you know that the darkest day of my life occurred. It was at 1:40 p.m. that my world became grossly dark, grossly dim, grossly sad. It was at that moment in time that Laurie Roth passed from this earth to heaven's doors.

There are no words to adequately express the depth of my sorrow right now. They say that the depth of your grief is precisely measured by the depth of your love. Having said that, there is no measurement for this, only emptiness. When you have been touched by an angel, you pray that you will always have her by your side. Unfortunately, that was not to be the case. Heaven had another idea. Despite all the other angels, heaven wanted this one back. I completely get that—I want her back too. And right now, my heart does not know what to do without the help of sweet Laurie Roth helping it beat.

What I do know is that Laurie is no longer in pain, no longer worried, no longer scared. She is free of the chains that tried to hold her back and never could. There will be no more chemo to hurt her, cancer to scare her, or scans to derail our lives. She is sitting up in heaven, living the good life with so many who loved her and went before her: her grandparents, my mom, Bryndahl, Hobiecat, Taylor, and Max.

And it is that image to which I will cling—the image of heaven's doors opening for the beautiful Laurie Roth and all our angels running toward her. Heaven's newest angel has already made it a more beautiful place.

How I go on without her is anyone's guess. I'm twelve hours out, and I have never felt more empty in my life. I was privileged to walk beside an amazing person who made me better just by being in my life. I learned so much from her grace, her strength, her courage. May I come to honor her by emulating even a fraction of who she was.

Good night, my angel. May you rest in peace, knowing that we are here missing you, loving you, waiting until the day when we meet again.

My Cardinal
April 22, 2013

Thank you for all of the love and support that you have showered on me through your calls, your texts, your posts, your cards, and your presence. Every time I looked up, another Lifesaver was walking up the driveway carrying food and drink in arms that were ready to hug me and hold me as I cried tears that I'm not sure will ever stop. You share my pain, my heartache, my loss. Our world will never be the same without beautiful Laurie to brighten it, make it funny, make it perfect.

I wake up every morning with the same thoughts: please let this have been a nightmare, please let her be here, please let me see her smile, hear her voice, hear that wonderful laugh one more time. I have selfishly wished her back a thousand times—not in the body she had near the end, but like she was as we knew her to be: strong, vibrant, amazing, and incredible. As I have said so many times, she deserved a better ending.

On the other hand, in many ways, Laurie simply got it right in fewer years than it takes most of us. Some of us will run it right up to the date stamp and never get it nearly as right as she did in fifty-one short years. How many more people could she make happy? In how many ways could she make this world better? How many more laughs and how much love could she bring to her sidekick? She did it all. She did it right. She did it perfectly.

Over the years, I have shared so many stories with Laurie. She always made me feel like the most interesting, fascinating, hilarious person in the room. She may have been doing the grocery list in her head or counting her teeth, but she always seemed to be rapt in my every word. Of all the talents she had, and she had countless, this one was particularly amazing.

A story I told her early on, I would like to tell now. I have had the privilege to live with some of the best people and pets that God created. I don't know how I keep lucking out, but I do. This story starts with my beloved Aunt Marion. She and my mom came to the States together from Prince Edward Island, Canada. They soon took the States by storm, these two stylish sisters with quick laughs and quicker wits. Like Laurie's, their fan clubs were huge, and I was the president of each.

After my dad passed and Aunt Marion got divorced, she came to live with Mom and me. She was with us for four hilariously fun years, but in the last year, she was diagnosed with colon cancer. A surgery showed that it was particularly aggressive, and chemo was not even recommended. They told us to take her home, enjoy the family, and find quality in her days. So home we went. Aunt Marion would sit at my mom's kitchen table, look out in the yard at the bird feeder, and say, "How I wish I could see a cardinal. I just think they are such beautiful birds." We ran all over trying to find the right seed to attract a cardinal, and not once did one come. Not once.

My aunt passed away, and our world was shaken upside down. This soul who had filled every corner of our home with so much love and fun was now gone. My mom lost her best friend and favorite sister in one fell swoop. To say that we were grieving was an understatement.

A few days after Aunt Marion's passing, Mom and I were sitting at her kitchen table. We were talking about how much we missed her, how empty life felt, how hurt our hearts were. I looked up and said, "Mom, look outside, look who's here." And there was a cardinal—a vibrantly red, absolutely gorgeous cardinal sitting and staring at us through the window. We knew Aunt Marion was safe, that her spirit would never leave us, and that she would come and visit us again.

My mom and I talked about how when others would pass in the family, it would the cardinal that would be the signal, the message back. So when I lost my beloved mom five years ago, I searched high and low for our message, a cardinal. A week went by, and nothing. I thought, "Mom forgot the signal." After a week and a half, I was so disheartened. Plus I was grieving the loss of her and how empty my world was. I woke up one morning and told Laurie that my heart was so heavy from missing my mom so much. We talked for a bit, and then Laurie said, "Lin, look out the window. Look across the street and see who's here." Across the street on our neighbor's front porch railing sat a vibrantly red, absolutely gorgeous cardinal. Never before had we seen one there, but it was a direct vision line into our living room, right to me crying on the couch. My mom hadn't forgotten the signal. In true Bert Jones fashion, she came in her own time, after all her reunions were over and the limbo stick had been put away.

The same thing happened with the loss of our eternal child, Max Jones, the cocker spaniel. When Maxie had some health issues a few years before he passed, I told him about the signal. He lived two more years and left us very suddenly early one morning, right here at home. Since he was as ding-a-lingy as a doorbell, I thought there was no way he would remember the signal. Oh, how I underestimated that boy. The day after he died, Laurie and I were bawling in the sunroom. Peter Pan was never to be in our arms again, and the hurt was far too much. Just then I looked up, and on the back fence, straight ahead of where we sat, perched a vibrantly red, absolutely gorgeous cardinal. Thank you, Maxie. You came back to your mommas right when we needed you the most.

You know where I'm going with this, right? Laurie passed at 1:40 p.m. on Friday. I bawled from that time until early morning before falling into a fitful sleep. I awoke to find that this wasn't just a nightmare, it was a nightmare from which I would never wake up to find a different outcome. While I was on the phone with my sister, completely inconsolable, I walked out to the sunroom just to be in the space of the house that Laurie loved so much. Tears were streaming down my face. I said to my sister, "I just miss her so much. I just want to see her one more time."

I looked out the sliding glass doors, and there sat a cardinal on our fence. A vibrantly red, absolutely gorgeous cardinal was staring right into my eyes, just like Laurie had done the day before when I let her go. The cardinal sat there, we locked eyes, and I knew Laurie was safe. I knew this signal was my message that my dear, sweet Laurie Roth was safe and at peace. Just as important, she was back with me, and oh, the comfort that came from seeing that beautiful cardinal.

Since then, I've seen cardinals in the strangest places. I've seen them in places where Laurie often looked for one but never saw one. I've seen them in places where Journey and Harbour and I are walking and a cardinal is near to us, flying past us, or waiting for us at the next turn. I've seen them in places where only Laurie would know that I would go as I stumble to put one foot in front of the other during these painful, painful days. My cardinal is back, and that brings peace to my heart. It's still broken, it still hurts, but knowing she's safe is all that I ever wanted for her.

Thank you for everything. We were touched by an angel. May we always, always feel her gentle, vibrantly red, absolutely gorgeous spirit all around us.

"I'm Here! I'm Here! I'm Here!"
May 1, 2013

I wanted to take some time to thank you for the amazing outpouring of support that you have shown to me and our family. In the midst of our darkest days, your love lifted us and enabled us to put one foot in front of the other. Just like you did for Laurie and me so many times, you were there for us every step of the way.

Laurie's and my journey over the past ten months was taken one scan, one step, one day at a time. There were times when getting through even one day was too tall an order. So we would reduce it down to the increments that we could manage—getting from one hour, one minute, even one second to another. The road that you walk with cancer as your very unwelcome companion is one that gives new meaning to fear, pain, and worry. But you have no other choice than to take the path you are given.

Laurie's Journey

And if you are my hero, you try to make the best of this awful situation.

And nobody did that better than Laurie. In the midst of all she was going through, her smile was ever present. When the scans did not reward her with good news, she was certainly disappointed, but she would turn her thoughts to more positive resolve. When her will and her might were tested beyond human response, she'd come out punching, come out fighting, come out the victor every time.

I refuse to use the phrase that Laurie "lost her battle to cancer." Nope, not going to say it. It may be semantics to some, but in my heart of hearts, Laurie Roth is a winner and always will be. This battle was not lost. Our champ took the path that she knew was best to take, and she won. She took her fight as far as she humanly could, and when she'd had enough, we locked eyes, we said goodbye, and she went to a whole new winner's circle. It was not the ending I wanted, but it was the ending she deserved. One that ends here and begins there. One that stops the hurt and brings her joy. One that allows her soul to sing.

We didn't have much singing around the house these past few months. I've always been prone to belt out a show tune at any given moment, often to Laurie's chagrin, but even those weren't heard too often recently. Laurie wasn't singing much either. Her energy was in survivor mode, not singing mode. But here's what I've noticed since Laurie passed: my girl is singing. Every single day, my cardinal comes to the fence right outside the sunroom, and every single day I hear that bird singing like nobody's business. It is music to my ears and a balm to my heart.

The cardinal has a distinct song. Having heard it and listened for it for years, I know it through and through. Laurie's seems just a bit different. Her song seems to say, "I'm here! I'm here! I'm here!" followed by a long happy whistle. There are other times when I think she's saying, "Don't give the dogs so many treats!" But that's probably just my guilty conscience from giving the dogs so many treats. At any rate, her song soothes me, just like Laurie's soft voice always did. Whether she's right in front of me or off in the distance, my girl is singing and telling me she's safe. She's telling me she's no longer hurting, no longer in pain, no longer worried. She's so darn happy that she's singing about it. And while I miss her more than words could ever say, and my heart is splintered in tiny, tiny pieces, hearing her sing again brings me pure joy.

I hope you hear our cardinal. When you do, you will also hear and have pure joy. It won't completely take the loss away; it won't completely mend your heart; it won't laugh at your ridiculous jokes or make you feel like you hung the moon every single day. But because we loved Laurie so much, we must have joy when she does. She earned the right to spend every second of every day living in pure joy. If it can't be here, then I am so glad it's there. My girl was pure joy on this earth. I am thankful she's been given pure joy forever.

Thank you again for all your love and support. You are pure joy to me, and I am so very thankful for each of you.

My Everything
May 12, 2013

A dear friend of ours, Margi, sent me a CD filled with songs that she said reminded her of Laurie and me. The second I heard the song "Everything" by Michael Bublé, I immediately thought of Laurie.

> *You're a falling star*
> *You're the getaway car*
> *You're the line in the sand when I go too far*
> *You're the swimming pool on an August day*
> *And you're the perfect thing to say . . .*
> *And in this crazy life*
> *And through these crazy times*
> *It's you, it's you*
> *You make me sing*
> *You're every line*
> *You're every word*
> *You're everything*

Laurie truly was my falling star. She truly was my getaway car. She quickly became my everything. And through all of our crazy times, it was always her. She was the constant in my life. She was the one who made the crazy days sane. We had a lot of those types of days, especially in the last few months. Our world felt like a snow globe that had been permanently turned upside down, and no matter how I tried, I couldn't get it to sit back up correctly. Then Laurie would rally, she'd get up again, and she would smile. And as the saying goes, all was right in my world. One person's beautiful smile can be that powerful. My one person's smile could turn my world upside *right*.

How I would love to see that smile right now. How I need that smile that warmed me to the core and always reminded me that things would be okay. When I shut my eyes, I still see Laurie's smile, that amazing, wonderfully warm smile. It would start with her mouth, crinkle up her nose, and end in those beautiful, joyful, peaceful eyes. It was like her face finished perfectly what her mouth so easily started. I always knew that when that smile came at me, I was the luckiest person in the universe. That smile meant joy, that smile meant safety, that smile meant my heart had landed right where it had longed to always be.

And it was infectious. Every single one of you know that I am right on this. If Laurie Roth smiled at you, it was game over. You were going to smile back no matter what. And not only that, her smile had a ripple effect that just kept on going. Like her life, one smile out of Laurie Roth brought countless smiles to others from others. I always told her that it was like her smile reached into my heart, squeezed it tight, and made me giddy. I had to smile back—no other response was even possible. It was the same with her laugh. Talk about infectious! Her laugh should be all of our ringtones—no phone would ever be answered again. We would just want to hear Laurie's beautiful and joyful laugh over and over again.

These past twenty-three days have brought a range of emotions to our house. My memories go to all different days—her last days, her very last day, the first day of waking up without her, and every day afterward that brings the realization that she's not here and won't be back. I make myself look at her picture, and while it makes me cry, it always makes me smile. Her smile beaming back at me creates the desired effect whether in person or in print. I make myself think of wonderful memories, which are countless. I think of us on the boat, taking drives, taking walks, enjoying the dogs, sitting in the sunroom or on our deck, enjoying our friends and our families. I'm so thankful for these memories because they bring her back to me, if only for a bit.

I make myself go to the sunroom door every morning to see if my cardinal is there. I'm usually there early in anxious anticipation.

Laurie's Journey

Laurie always bordered on the tardy side, and I always waited her out. Her tardiness never caused us to be late, but God love her, she could run our departure time right up to the last minute. I am the opposite. I like to leave a little early, maybe even arrive a little early; at the very least, I like to believe that we will get out the door and arrive on time. But nagging is annoying, and it really only results in bogging the whole process down. So we developed a five-minute rule: if I was ready to go, I couldn't encourage her to get going unless five minutes had passed with Laurie appearing not to be any more ready than when the five minutes started. I have no idea how this practice began. My bet is that it's an elementary school teacher trick, like giving an annoying child busywork to keep her out of your hair. Needless to say, I fell for it every time. So now is no different. I give her the five-minute rule, and without fail, every single day since she has passed, up she comes. This lone, vibrantly red, gorgeous cardinal, singing long before I see it, gracefully arrives on our fence and makes my day complete. We lock eyes, we stare at each other for a long time, she sings a bit, and off she goes.

I'll take it. It gives my heart the exact right kick-start that it needs each morning. It makes me smile, and sometimes it even makes me laugh. Sometimes Laurie is singing so much, it's like she drank way too much and is just belting out tune after tune. I'm beginning to think that heaven has quite a nightclub, because Laurie is still feeling the effects by the time she arrives here in the morning. Seeing her, locking eyes with her—well, it is exactly the connection I need from her, right when I need it the most. Like she always did, she starts my day with her beautiful presence, her smile, and our connection. Our hearts can't be divided, and for that, I am so very grateful. And while missing her weighs my heart down to immeasurable levels on most days, her pure love and joy never fail to bring my heart to a better place. She always has and always will. She was my everything then and is my everything now. I am blessed.

And thank you to all of you for bringing my heart to a better place. Your love and care and support continue now like they have since the first step of this journey. We were not alone then, and I'm not alone now. The army continues to circle the wagons and hold me close in hugs and love. Thank you, army. Thank you from the bottom of my very grateful heart. I love each of you.

Connected
May 19, 2013

I just wanted to check in and thank you again for your continued love and support. As you can well imagine, these continue to be dark, harsh days filled with much emotion and far too much reality—reality that reminds me that my girl isn't here, that I won't hear her voice or hear that beautiful laugh. It is a reality that I never, ever wanted. It is a reality that hurts to the core and seems to break my heart into more pieces.

It has been a time of many emotions. There are times that make me smile, and times when my mind can't pull the happy memories up fast enough before replacing one with another. We had so many good times and fun times and happy times that it would seem that whenever my heart gets sad again, all it should have to do is rewind the tape, hit "play," and relive our beautiful life.

Ah, but there's the rub—right now all I want is to relive my life with Laurie. I don't want to do this road without her. I want to relive it with Laurie right beside me, enjoying it and making plans to make new memories together. I want her on the couch with me as we replay the home movies of our one and only beautiful life. I want her to help put my Humpty Dumpty heart back together again.

But it's not to be, and my heart simply doesn't know where to sit. I tell myself to be patient with myself. That it's only been a month, I say. Actually, today is the thirtieth day that we have been apart. For two people who never spent more than forty-eight hours apart, thirty days is forever. Thirty-one won't be any picnic either. Even when I will come to count our days apart in years, not days, every increment will have that same surreal feel to it.

We weren't designed to be apart. Laurie and I were two pieces of the puzzle that fit perfectly. Our hearts were home and our lives completed each other. We had a deep connection tying soul to soul. It is exactly that deep connection that helps keep me going today. It helped keep me going yesterday and the twenty-eight days before. And I pray it will keep me going until I see my girl again.

That connection comes in a cardinal on my fence every single morning singing her tunes. That connection comes when the tears stream down my face and a cardinal comes and lands in a tree in our yard where I've never seen one before—but it's the tree that I happen to be facing, and after hearing a little tune, I look up and see that gorgeous bird sitting there, staring at me, locked on me. That connection comes in a cardinal that finds Journey, Harbour, and me in all our new places, leading us down new paths, singing and flying and swooping so close I can hear the wings as they flutter. Connected beyond words.

After I managed to weasel my way into Laurie's heart, she told me that she always knew I was out there for her, and she knew that someday she would find me. She said, "Now that I've found you, I'm never letting you go." When the dark days of our journey began to rear their ugly head, we had some very emotional conversations, ones that a sidekick and her hero never wanted to have. But we knew we had to. It was in one of those conversations that my girl told me, "I will never, ever let you go. I will come back and find you somehow. We are that connected." Always true to her word, she hasn't let me go, she has come back to find me, and we are that connected.

Her spirit is in every fiber of my bones and every corner of my soul. Some days it hurts to know I will only ever have her in spirit. But on most days, it is soothing to me and often my greatest source of comfort. Her spirit is as peaceful and gentle and graceful as Laurie herself was. Her spirit lifts my heart, helps dry my tears, and helps me take the baby steps to tomorrow. She is always with me, always finding me—we are that connected.

My connection to you soothes my soul as well. You grieve with me; you loved Laurie deeply too; you miss her and her beautiful smile. You share with me that a cardinal came to you too, and it brings me incredible comfort to know that she is making her rounds. She loved each of you so much, and her spirit remains in you too. It won't always feel like enough, but if you close your eyes and take a deep breath, Laurie's beautiful spirit will do the rest. It always did, it always has, and it always will.

Thank you for all of your love to me and the Golden Girls. We so appreciate your prayers and your support. This is an amazing army, and we love each of you so deeply.

Memorial Day
May 27, 2013

I'll be honest with you, I was kind of dreading Memorial Day. Although it is a day designed to honor men and women who died in the armed services, we have broadened it to be a day to honor all those who have passed. Knowing that, I had this sense of dread—this utter apprehension of this one day. I was downright fearful for it to arrive. And then it was like a light went off in my pea brain and a voice inside me said, "You honor her every day. Monday will not be any different." Since the little voice was right on target, it clearly could not be mine. I'm guessing it's my mother again—she's usually right on the money in all things Linda Jones.

So the dread faded, the apprehension dropped, and the fear never made it to fruition. Every day is a day to honor Laurie—to honor her beautiful soul, which graced my life and made me better, certainly made my world better, and gave me the most wonderful reason to open my eyes every morning. Immediately upon waking, I always knew it would be a good day because she was in it. We would share the day, share our lives, share our love. It truly doesn't get any better than that.

Laurie used to marvel at how happy I was right when I woke up. As similar as we were, we were different in our morning rituals. She liked to ease into a morning. After a few cups of coffee and getting some things in her routine under her belt, she hit the day at full speed. But it wasn't right out of the box. She had a cautious approach to the day until she hit her stride—after that there was absolutely no stopping her. Then there was me. I would wake up whistling, much to Laurie's chagrin, and often I was talking and singing, a combo that is admittedly annoying. I was absolutely giddy about greeting the day. There were even a few times when Laurie would look at me, smile that gorgeous smile, and say, "Chuckles, could you take it down a notch or twelve for just a few minutes?"

I couldn't help it. I am naturally hardwired for happiness. My perfume is Happy by Clinique. My blood type is B positive. (Get it? Be positive? I'm not kidding.) Our closet is filled with every "Life is good" shirt ever made. Every glass is half full in my cupboard. I am just a cockeyed optimist at heart. Life is usually going to land in a really good place in my world. To prove it, after I was transferred to Bloomington, Illinois, thinking I'd be here eighteen months tops, I ended up meeting and sharing my life with the most beautiful person on earth and never leaving. It doesn't get any better than that.

So what does a cockeyed, whistling optimist do when life gets as bad as it did thirty-eight days ago? My sense of who I innately am has been significantly challenged and questioned and downright bullied by the reality that my life is forever changed. The other half of my soul no longer wakes up with me. My right arm, my right hand, my right everything is all wrong, because Laurie is not there. There's an echo now where my heartbeat used to go out and return with Laurie's. It simply doesn't beat the same and never will. Who I am is not who I was, and part of me never, ever will be that person again.

But even on days when my heart feels like it is splintered into far too many pieces, when I can't see anything because there are only tears in my eyes, when even a baby step seems far too big a leap—even during all of that, I know that I was so very privileged to share this road with Laurie. Having the honor of being her sidekick is by far the best present that I have ever unwrapped. To have had her in my life, to have heard her laugh every day, to have had her smile at me not just once, but countless times—now, that's livin', folks. That's what life is all about.

Laurie's Journey

If you get really lucky, you find your one true thing—the very thing that makes you tick and keeps you tickled, that soothes your soul and hangs the moon, that keeps you hardwired for happiness even when the days get dark and the road gets long and the ending is not your "happily ever after."

So that's what I cling to: the fact that I got so very lucky. I won the lottery of life when I met Laurie. We had a life that, in our opinion, was extraordinary. We cherished the gift that we had been given. We carved out a magical life that made us both so incredibly happy. Long before we knew the days were numbered, we never took one day for granted. Not one.

And because of that, I have a boatload of wonderful memories that will help take me across the shore from the life we had to the one I'm reluctantly starting now. I have this beautiful spirit that sits right in my heart, and when I stop crying and start listening, I hear Laurie's sweet voice reminding me that nothing can divide us. Not time, not space, not death. We may be divided physically, but our spirits are sewn tightly together.

As a reminder, I have a cardinal that comes to the fence every single morning, locks eyes with me, shares a few minutes of my day, and makes me smile. And when I smile, it's my old smile. It's the one I used to wake up with. It's the one that made me sing and whistle. It is this old smile that makes me think that maybe, just maybe, I might even wake up and whistle again. Whistling will come. And much to your chagrin, so will my singing. Right now, I'll just take the baby steps, the cardinals, and the smiles. Because right now, it truly doesn't get better than that.

Thank you for filling the gaps. You fill me up with love and support. You truly are lifesavers—always have been, always will be. It's who you are. I love you all.

Ordinary Days
June 5, 2013

Just checking in and letting you know that your love and support help more than words could possibly convey properly. As you always have, you come in cards and emails, texts and calls. You come in the form of invites for breakfast, lunch, and dinner. You come, you sit, and you let me cry or laugh or babble on about our girl. The bottom line is that you were here with Laurie and me, and now you are here for me and the Golden Girls. Our lives have changed in a very major way, but the familiarity of your love is an amazing comfort.

Speaking of familiarity, shortly after Laurie passed, someone said to me that "it will be the ordinary things that get ya." I listened politely and yet had no idea what this person was talking about. After all, at that time, nothing seemed ordinary—everything seemed foreign. It was if I had been dropped into another country, or possibly another planet, where very few things looked or felt familiar. Ordinary means normal, customary, routine, constant. The second Laurie left this world, ordinary seemed to leave with her. My normal, customary routine had come to a screeching halt, and my constant was no longer here.

That's what deep grief does. At least it has done that to me. It takes your normal life, turns it upside down, and refuses to put it right side up again. Sleep eludes you, tears follow you everywhere, and you simply don't know your own life anymore. Actually, you are very worried that you *do* know your own life—that this hole in your heart, the silence in your head, the "hello" you put out that will never be returned by the one voice you long to hear, really is your life now. It's the life you never wanted, but it's here because of the ending that you were forced to face.

Then one day you reach for the phone to call Laurie from work because she will just crack up at this story you have to tell her. Another day, while reading the paper, you finish a section and go to hand it over to her and trade for the section that she just finished. You wake up and say "Good mornin', Sunshine!" and nobody groans in return and begs you to use your inside voice and use it about ten houses down. Yep. It's the ordinary things that get ya.

It was the ordinary things I loved—every single one of them. We had so many fun times, so many laughs, so many wonderful conversations, more often than not about nothing. Laurie and I could take nothing and make it something that we both would enjoy again and again. And I cherish each and every one of those absolutely-about-nothing times. We were in each other's pockets, carrying each other around in our hearts, and when we were apart, we longed to be together again. It was our regular old routine, with its very regular rhythm, that allowed our life to be oh so very remarkable for us. Carving out this ordinary path with this absolutely extraordinary person was all I ever wanted.

And while it is the ordinary things that will "get ya"—and trust me, they have and they will again—I'm finding that there is comfort in those regular ol' days that brought about the ordinary memories that we made. I cherished them then, and I cherish them now. I never needed cancer to bully me into appreciating the beautiful soul with whom I was blessed to share my life. Nope. I knew it from the start. I knew that if Laurie Roth would bring me into her world, mine would be complete. I knew that we would spend ordinary days living out extraordinary dreams. And that we did. And for that, I am eternally grateful.

So come and get me, ordinary things. Get me and always remind me that the little things Laurie and I did add up to some of the best times of our life together. Play our highlight reel again and again, always reminding me that the magic grew from the smallest of events and brought about the largest of joys. Never let me forget that sitting on the deck with Laurie, watching the dogs play or the cats fight or the people on the trail go by in their anything-but-ordinary outfits, that these are the times to cherish. That when you can be with someone and not say one single word, but convey all that you want to express in a look, a smile, or a heartbeat, then you have been given a remarkable gift. That I was. I was given an amazing gift who simply can't stop giving. Her spirit finds me, it locks in, and it brings the comfort I need right then and there.

Many of you had those memorable, seemingly ordinary, but amazingly remarkable moments with Laurie too. I've heard so many stories that start with "one time Laurie and I were just sitting there" and end with a marvelous, often hilarious, never-to-be-forgotten moment. She did that. She did that so very effortlessly. She brought you into her world, life unfolded, fun happened, and you were and are all the better for it. I know I am. Cherish those ordinary times, because I promise you, they will bring you extraordinary joy, extraordinary love, and extraordinary comfort. Laurie Roth can do it no other way.

Heal, Journey, Heal
June 18, 2013

Many of you have been so kind to ask for an update on how the pets are doing through this time. You know how integral they were to Laurie and she was to them. The love they shared wasn't severed at death, any more than mine with Laurie has been, or yours. Like us, pets form deep bonds with the humans who share their lives. Those pets who have been lucky enough to live under

Laurie's Journey

our roof found heaven on earth thanks to Laurie's loving care. How they wish, like all of us, that their mama could come back and turn their world upside right again. And none of our pets wish that more than sweet Journey.

Journey and Laurie have their own love story. We met Journey when she was about three and a half weeks old. She was a beautiful little butterball who stole our hearts immediately. But it was Laurie with whom Journey fell most madly in love. The feeling was so mutual. From the minute they met, they were head over heels in love with each other. Not too many days passed without us popping over to see those gorgeous puppies. I'd be picking up one after the other, trying to get my fill of puppy breath, snuggling them close, cuddling all of them. I'd look over and there would be Laurie, holding the same pup the entire time: Journey. I'm shocked that Journey ever learned to walk properly, since she never needed the use of her legs with Laurie around. We would walk in and Laurie would swoop her up, hold her close, kiss her countless times, and whisper sweet nothings in her ear. I'd try to hand her a different puppy to enjoy, and Laurie would smile sweetly at it but never let go of Journey. They both knew that was the plan: Mama never letting go of Journey, and Journey never letting go of Mama.

Their love grew from their initial meeting at three and a half weeks and every day thereafter. They enjoyed the simple things, fun things, learning new things. They trained in obedience, in the sport of rally, and in agility. They were beautiful to watch, each knowing each other's move and what should come next. It was pure love in motion. Journey locked on Laurie, watching her so closely, waiting for the next signal. The signal could come with a slight move of Laurie's finger or hand, or maybe just the intonation of Laurie's voice. Journey knew them all, anticipated some, and anxiously awaited others. They were a dynamic duo no matter what they did—completely focused on each other, oblivious to anyone else around. And at the end of every class, every run, and every competition, they would celebrate like they had won the Westminster Dog Show! Journey would jump up into Laurie's arms, and Laurie would beam and carry her around, never letting her go. It was a perfect picture of happiness every single time.

Obedience training came easily to them. Since I had never really known what it meant to have a dog that obeyed, I marveled at how easy Journey and Laurie made it look. Admittedly, Max and I had been essentially kicked out of puppy obedience class due to both of our behavior issues (we had little pride and had also been kicked out of better places, so it had little impact on either one of us). I smugly left the building, Max prancing at my side, almost *appearing* obedient. He wasn't. Instead, Peter Pan was anxious to get to the car so we could get over to Dairy Queen for his ice cream cone. I'm not kidding.

Anyway, Journey and Laurie burned up the obedience classes. Journey loved learning, and there was no better teacher than Laurie, whether you had two feet or four feet. Whatever command Laurie gave, Journey would happily do. She loved to please Laurie, and she loved the sense of routine. It didn't hurt that Max ran this house like a German clock shop—he ate at 7:00 a.m. and 4:30 p.m., on the nose. There were treats dispensed at hourly intervals in between or whenever he demanded, and his walks came an hour after each meal. If you veered from this routine, he let you know—loudly and often. So even though I believe that Journey is hardwired to comply, she had it reinforced by the little general she grew up with.

Laurie's Journey

In no time, she could sit, stay, lie down, roll over—the list went on and on. But of all the commands she learned, Journey's personal favorite was "heel." When Laurie said "Heel, Journey, heel," then Journey got to be right by Mama's side. This command seemed inherent to Journey. After all, we didn't call her "Velcro" for nothing—she couldn't get close enough to Laurie! The heel command was a match made in heaven for those two. The only part of obedience training that Journey didn't like was when she had to sit and stay while Laurie left her sight. Journey's heart would grow heavy, and she would whine and cry. That one minute when Laurie was out of her sight was the longest minute of Journey's life. Her heart beat better, stronger, and happier when Laurie was in her sight. How I understand that.

And when Laurie got sick, Journey came to know the good days from the not-so-good. She knew when Mom needed her to just sit by her side, and she knew when a walk might do us all good. She knew when Mom should rest, and she knew when it was okay to play. She knew her mom through and through—so much so that this sweet little soul also knew when things were going south. About four days before Laurie passed, Journey began wanting to spend more time, almost all of her time, in the garage. Please keep in mind that Journey and Harbour are not garage dogs. They are sofa dogs, they are sunroom dogs, they are lie-on-the-chaise-lounge-on-the-deck dogs. So I can assure you, the garage is not where they typically like to be. But Journey was sensing something that was too hard to face, and like all of us, she could barely stand to watch.

At bedtime on those four nights, I had to coax Journey into the house. She would reluctantly come in but didn't really want to be in the bedroom. The very place where her favorite person was, she didn't want to be. This kept up for four solid days, until approximately twenty minutes before Laurie passed. Just as I was about to start talking Laurie into leaving, just as I was about to ask her to make one decision purely for herself, just as I was about to ask the other half of my heart to take hers somewhere safe, Journey scratched on the bedroom door to come in. I knew that she knew. I knew she had to be there. I knew that she had come to say goodbye.

So in she came—so very brave, so very strong, so very sad. In front of me and the hospice nurse, Journey hopped up on the bed, like she had done a thousand times before. This time she took a long look in Laurie's eyes, kissed her on the forehead, and lay down right by her side. She was more settled than I had seen her in four long days. Laurie knew she was there and seemed more settled too. As I talked and Laurie listened, Journey just lay there. Another faithful sidekick, another adoring fan, another soul mate letting go. And when Laurie left us, Journey got up, kissed her again, gently stepped over her, and lay down on the other side of her. It would take a few of us to coax her down off the bed about an hour and a half later. Journey knew what I knew—there was not a better place on earth than by Laurie's side. It would be hard to give that up. In fact, it has proven to be near impossible for both of us.

This past Friday, it was eight weeks since we let our girl go. Like me, Journey is trying to figure out our new normal. Try as I might, few things hold the same fun, the same adventure, the same love as they did before. We tried to go to the cabin where we like to spend our weekends, but Journey didn't want to get out of the truck. She eventually did, bless her heart, but reluctantly. We managed to stay only about fifteen minutes, and leaving was as much my idea as it was Journey's. The one we always had with us, the one who made every bit of our world complete, the one who made that cabin all that it is, wasn't there. It didn't seem right to be there without her. It doesn't seem right to be anywhere without her.

It is a long, rough road without the other half of your soul. I see that in the eyes that look back at me in the mirror every day. And I see that in the eyes of Laurie's other soul mate, Journey. I've tried to follow the routines that Laurie set. We try to keep busy and go on long walks and longer drives. We try and we try and we try. But pain doesn't go away because of a long walk or a good, long drive or eating at the same time you've always eaten. The one you loved the very most is not here, and it hurts. There is simply no way around that.

That is not to say that Journey doesn't love me. I know she does. I'm the pushover mom who can be talked into anything, primarily belly rubs on demand and kisses as often as are wanted. I'm the protector mom that she would run to when the other mom had shampoo in one hand and bath towels in the other. I'm the one who never, ever will make Journey do one single thing that she doesn't want to do. In short, Laurie was Alpha and I was Omega, and it worked really, really well in this house. Journey is missing her Alpha and hanging close to her Omega, and we're all praying that the second in command, Alicat, doesn't take control. Heaven help us all if that happens.

And then there's Harbour. Journey and I could both learn a lot from her. Harbour loved Laurie very deeply too. But this old soul seems to understand the circle of life. She shows Journey and me that you should take one day at a time, no faster or slower than what you can handle. In doing so, you find you land safely—maybe still sadly, but safely—in the next day. With any luck, you arrive with just a little more strength that day so that you have the energy to enjoy some of it. And you keep on building one day upon the other, blessed to have shared your life with this incredible person, missing her, but knowing she's safe. Until Journey and I fully learn this lesson, Harbour sticks close to us, loving us through it as only that gentle soul can do. Thank you, Missy Harbour.

Like me, like all of us, Journey will eventually find her way. Together, she and I will get through this. Together, we will all get through this. I remind Journey of what her mom taught her so many years ago, the command that came so easily then and that I pray will come very soon. It's a little twist on Laurie's words, but a command all the same: Heal, Journey, heal. Feel your mom's spirit and let her heal your heart. She is right beside you, all around you, tucked right inside your soul. Even when you can't see her, feel her, or touch her, her love remains. She would want nothing more than for you to heal, sweet Journey, heal. Amen.

I so appreciate the continued love and support that all of you shower down upon us. You are an amazing comfort to us as we work each day to find our way without our girl. Thank you for standing beside us, loving us, and praying for us to heal.

The Song Remembers When
July 7, 2013

Someone recently asked me what has been the hardest part of the past eleven weeks. The question actually got me thinking—no easy feat with this noggin. I realized that there are many answers to this question, all very dependent on the day, the hour, the minute in which I may be asked.

Laurie's Journey

There are common themes, though, to the past eleven weeks. My heart isn't right, breathing isn't right, walking upright isn't right. My heart feels like at least half of it is gone, and the part that remains is splintered into tiny, heavy pieces. My chest feels like it has a five-hundred-pound gorilla on it, and my guess is that his name is Grief. And Grief isn't showing any signs of getting off anytime soon. My feet know they have to take steps, baby ones and backward ones and sometimes even forward ones. But where I am walking is not where I want to go. I'm on a path to my "new normal," and I'm not ready to face that reality. I'm not ready, and I don't want to.

While all of that is so very difficult, those are emotions and reactions and feelings that I expected. I knew it would be almost impossible to walk out of Camelot without my soul mate. I knew that going from paradise found to paradise lost would be about as devastating as it gets. I knew that giving up heaven on earth so that Laurie could have heaven forever would smash my heart to bits. This is pain that I'm not sure you ever recover from. You may learn to manage it a bit better, but get over it? Nah. Not even possible.

But it's the out-of-the-blue moments that knock me down just as fast as the moments I knew were coming. It's opening a drawer and seeing a card from Laurie that she snuck under my pillow a few months before she passed—a card that made me smile then and makes me cry now.

It's walking through the grocery store and grabbing the type of coffee that Laurie always drank, or the cookies she loved, or bananas with just the amount of ripeness that she always liked best. It's reaching for that "something" she loved and realizing that I will never buy anything for her again.

It is the unexpected times that shake your soul like a rag doll. You see, I'm just OCD enough to have a drawer for cards from Laurie to me, a drawer for cards from me to Laurie, and a whole other drawer for cards from all of you to both of us. Laurie and I loved to surprise each other with cards in different places, with yellow sticky notes in the toothpaste drawer, with notes taped to the steering wheel. We were two people who never took each other for granted, loving the surprise of a card or even a plain ol' sticky note. We have countless ones in their appropriate drawers.

The card I found last week was not in the proper drawer with the other cards. Why it was in the drawer where I found it, I have no idea. But seeing it, reading it, holding it—well, that's the stuff that brings me to my knees.

We both loved music. And like many people, we had special songs that meant something to us. They were "our songs." Until last week, I had not heard any of them since Laurie passed. Then, there I was, driving down the road and switching from one radio station to another, when I heard one of those songs starting. Immediately the tears filled my eyes, ran down my cheeks, and put everyone driving anywhere near me in grave danger (well, more so than usual). I couldn't see a thing as the song played through. I finally pulled into a parking lot and bawled my eyes out.

It was a beautiful song titled "The Song Remembers When." It's sung by Tricia Yearwood, and the first verse tells exactly how I felt that day. The song remembers—it remembers when we first heard it, where we were, and why it was ours. I remember when we sang it together, wrote parts of it to each other in our cards, and reminded each other how it fit us to a T. And as the song made me remember those times with Laurie, I wanted each and every one of them back. As I listened to that song, I missed her even more than I had before, and I am sure a dam broke in my heart . . . again.

That's the dance I'm in. I think that's the dance that is universal to grief, and I know many of you know this dance or have known it. There are memories that burn and hurt and bring a whole new rawness to an already gaping wound. Memories can be a healing balm, or they can open the wounds right back up again. In fact, they can border on both—a salve and a sore. But you know what? I wouldn't give any of them up. Not the painful ones, and not the peaceful ones. They must all appear, I must soak them in, and I must remember that each of them played a part in the amazing journey I was given with Laurie.

Because of Laurie Roth, I know that you can walk into a dog park, chase down an ill-behaved little cocker spaniel, and find the love of your life. I know that one person can truly be the difference maker in your life, the perfect hostess for your heart, and the one who will forever change you just by loving you. I know that you can make a promise that nothing will ever divide your love from this person. You can promise to have and to hold, to take this person in sickness and in health, right up until death do you part and beyond.

You can do all of this because you have a love that knows no limits. Laurie's and my love is not cut off at the boundary line between heaven and earth. The pearly gates can't keep us apart. We made good on our promise to each other to weave our souls together. While the pain in my soul is deep right now, my soul is better because of Laurie and the love she gave me. This connection is what ultimately soothes me. It is this love that carries me through the pain, through the sleepless nights, through the song remembering when.

It is the same for all of you who loved her. I hear the hurt in your voice and see the pain in your eyes when you talk about her, email me about her, text me that you miss her. Thank you for loving her that deeply. Please know that she loved you deeply too. We may be divided from her physically, but her love is woven inside us. Remember her smile that lit up a room, that great laugh that made you laugh just because you heard hers, and those warm and soulful eyes that brought peace and grace to your heart. The memories may hurt, but they help bring peace—night after night, day after day, baby step after baby step.

May my heart, may your heart, may the hearts of our Golden Girls begin to fill with Laurie's beautiful spirit, so that when the song remembers when, when our hearts are far too heavy, when the sound of her gentle voice is the only sound that will soothe, we will reach into our souls and find her there—find her nestled in, warming us from the inside out, bringing us peace as only sweet Laurie Roth could ever do. That is my solemn prayer for each of us. Amen.

In Honor
July 24, 2013

So we passed the three-month mark. Three months ago last Friday, my girl left this earth. Unbelievable, isn't it? This beautiful spirit that I never saw myself living without has now been gone for three months. Thirteen weeks and five days, to be exact. Who's counting? Me. Every day I count. Every day I cry. Every single day I wake up and talk myself into getting up.

She left too early for all of us, but perfectly timed for her, and that is all that matters. I truly believe that Laurie got it right. She got it right sooner than most of us, better than anyone I know.

Laurie's Journey

She so deserved to be free of the pain of this world, the fear of what else might be coming down the pike, free from the chains of cancer. I refuse to ever say that Laurie "lost her battle." I prefer to picture cancer swinging its nasty, mean arms at Laurie and getting nothing but air. Gotcha, cancer. My girl got the last one in on you. She took the hardest chemos, the harshest treatments, the hardest roads, and steered herself straight up to heaven. No way did Laurie lose. Uh-uh. Folks, she won.

And when she walked away from cancer as the winner, she also won a lot more. She won the golden ticket to eternal life. She won the right to fly in and out of our lives as a beautiful cardinal who sings to me every single day. She won the battle here so she can spread her spirit everywhere. She won. And that was all I ever wanted. One thing that this long road has taught me is that you can't have it both ways. You can't keep her safe and keep her here. Loving her to pieces isn't going to keep the wolf from banging down your door. So you keep her safe, you love her to pieces, and you let her go.

It's no secret that Laurie hung the moon for me. I doubt she set out to be my hero, but in a blink of an eye, she did it. It wasn't how she faced cancer that gave her that moniker. Nope. Cancer simply highlighted and showcased her hero status. Of all the nicknames I ever gave her, "Hero" came about early in our game. Like my mom, Laurie became my hero because of how she lived her life. She lived her life as gently and as sweetly as I have ever seen it done. She gave people passes for not-such-great behavior. She turned the other cheek so many times, she should have had a permanent kink in her neck. She paid it forward every chance she got.

When you were around Laurie Roth, your blood pressure dropped. Did you ever notice that? It wasn't coincidence. It wasn't medicine. It wasn't anything but that gentle soul working her magic on you. She spoke quietly and sweetly and kindly. She held your heart in her hands, and you felt so darn safe that you never wanted it to end. How I know and remember and miss that feeling. I told her that I was in awe of how she treated people. I told her, "You know, we're all supposed to do that, but few of us get it right." She just laughed, shrugged me off, and refused to think that she was doing anything out of the ordinary. She was right. It wasn't out of the ordinary for Laurie Roth!

So here I am, thirteen weeks and five days into living my life without my girl beside me. My sleepless nights give me a lot of time for deep thought—well, thoughts as deep as this simpleton can muster. But on one such night, when I was especially lost, Laurie came and reminded me of how I could find my way.

She always thought that if we could all be just a little bit nicer, a little bit kinder, a little bit more understanding, then how nice and kind and understanding this world might be. She always thought it was worth a shot. I always agreed with her. I always made half-hearted attempts to follow her lead. I failed miserably. But I'd come home, observe my shining example of being the change we need to see in this world, and get up and try it again. Laurie always complimented my attempts—the teacher through and through. Even when the student fails, find something (in my case, anything) to compliment.

But on that particular sleepless night, I vowed that I would really try to be better, to be kinder, to be sweeter. And as with all my previous vows to her, I know I have to make this one stick. How better to honor Laurie than by trying to emulate her beautiful life? How better to recognize her gentleness than by being more gentle to others myself? What better tribute could I offer to my girl than, next time I get cut off on Veterans Parkway, not throwing hand signals like I'm a gangbanger? I only wish I was kidding.

I have a long way to go to make this attitude a part of my everyday life. Like all of us, I can be nice, I can be kind, I can be tolerant. Yet there are more days than I care to admit when I choose to be not so nice, not so kind, and not even one bit tolerant. Here's the problem now: I no longer have my sweet sounding board waiting at home to talk me off the ledge. My patient listener is not there to always remind me that "he didn't mean it the way he said it," that "people are inherently good, they just have bad days," that "your lack of the extra ketchup you asked for on your Happy Meal cheeseburger is not the end of the world." I'm not so sure about the last one, but I'm with Laurie on the other two.

Working to honor my girl this way serves a twofold purpose. I might actually become nicer (a bonus for all of you fine people!). And it keeps her even closer to me. I didn't even think that was possible. But I've noticed that when I'm kinder, I feel her spirit within me. When I'm nicer, I feel her love filling me up all over again. When a guy whips in front of me on Vernon Avenue and makes me burn up my brakes, I feel her arm holding mine back from whaling on the horn. It's a beautiful thing. It's a wonderful way to try to take my baby steps. It's living like Laurie would have me do. It might just work. If nothing else, as Laurie always said, it's worth a shot.

Also, so many of you have asked about Journey that I wanted to give a quick update. I think she's a pinch better. The cabin is still not her favorite place, she still whines at the bedroom door every so often, and there are still more days than not when her precious eyes reflect her little broken heart. But last week, she actually played in the backyard. That, my friends, was a major breakthrough. During the hottest week of the summer, Journey decided that playing outside again would be fun. And even though it felt like we were three inches from the sun, I couldn't pass this up.

We had a lot of fun. Journey was wagging and barking and rolling around like the little nut that she often showed Laurie and I that she could be. It was music to my soul to see this little spirit enjoying her backyard and toys again. Then, as if we both remembered at the same time, while I was kneeling down by her, petting and praising her, she tucked her head into my chest. This is an old favorite move of Journey's. It is done when she needs comfort, when she needs loving, when she needs to cry a bit. So cry we did. Not just a bit, but a lot. She kept her head tucked safely in my chest for almost ten minutes. Her head was wet with my tears. It was a good cry for both of us.

And guess who joined us? Yep—up in the best branch for a bird's-eye view sat our cardinal. As Journey and I were crying, we heard the song of our girl. I looked up and there she sat, staring down, singing her heart out. I told Journey that Mom was watching us and loving us and comforting us. I know Journey felt her too. We began playing again, and that cardinal watched us the whole time. She finally flew off when Journey headed for the door. It was a banner night—Journey played and our cardinal watched. It felt like old times—old times that we all so desperately needed.

So, army, thank you. May you know that the kindness and thoughtfulness and love that you have always shown have made such impression on me, a difference for me, a softer landing for this fall. I have been surrounded by angels every step of the way, and I appreciate each one of you. May I come even close to somehow paying your love forward. May I be the light on someone's dark road that you have been for me. It would appear that you learned Laurie's life lesson long before I did—no surprise there. From the bottom of my grateful heart, thank you.

Love Always Wins

So that's our story. It certainly did not have the ending we hoped for. As two people who found the extraordinary love that most only dream of, we believed we were living a fairy tale. A beautiful hero and her faithful sidekick were living life attached at the heart. All we ever wanted was a "happily ever after" ending. Sadly, we didn't get it. Instead, we were forced to make good on the vow we prayed would come long down our road: until death do us part.

Death does part us. It divides us. It separates us. No two ways around it, it absolutely does. The one left behind is broken with a void that will never, ever be filled. But here is what I have discovered: we are separated only physically. In the time that Laurie has been gone, I have found that she is still deep within me, all around me, a part of me. I close my eyes and see her beautiful and beaming smile. I listen and still hear her sweet and gentle voice. I rest and find her in my dreams, waiting for me, smiling at me, reminding me that she is safe.

She is my inner core, my secret thoughts, the other half of my heart. Our souls are stitched together with seams of timeless love and deep devotion that death can neither conquer nor separate. The bottom line is that death doesn't get the last say. As our minister said at Laurie's celebration of life service, love gets the last say. Love wins. Love always wins. I'm living proof that yes, it does.

Made in the USA
Lexington, KY
28 February 2014